ADVENTURE ON

FINESSING ADVENTURE TO DRIVE KICK-ASS DIABETES DOMINATION

ERIN SPINETO

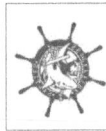

SEA PEPTIDE PUBLISHING

CALIFORNIA PROMISES
Copyright © 2022 Erin Spineto

For Information, Contact:
Sea Peptide Publishing
Carlsbad, CA, 92011
www.SeaPeptide.com

ISBN-13: 978-0-9882065-4-0
Second Edition: August 2022

To Tony,

For putting up with all my wild adventures.

CONTENTS

READ ME

FIRST

I am so excited to start this journey with you. I'm sure in buying this book you already have felt a little motivation stirring.

As you continue in this book, I will bring you through the process of adventure, from inception to execution. There are four parts to this challenge, Dream, Plan, Train, and Execute, each focusing on a different aspect of the process. Each part will provide you with instruction, ideas, inspiration, and tips to make your journey a little easier.

But to get the most out of this process, it is important that you really invest in it; invest in yourself. Adventure will do amazing thing for you, but it won't do anything without some time and effort on your part.

Think deeply about each part. Really dig into what you are made of, what you enjoy, and what you are capable of. The more you invest in this process, the more you will get out of it.

If you are looking to dig deeper, there are reflection questions for each chapter in the free workbook at www.SeaPeptide.com/adventureonworkbook .

So let's dream. And then let's plan, train, and execute our adventures. We can share our tales along the way so we can be inspired by each other. I am excited to see what you come up with. And get ready for this moment to be something that you will look back on as a real turning point in your life.

Now, let's look at why adventure works so well...

LINKS IN THIS BOOK

All of the research articles and links to other platforms in this book can be found organized by chapter at www.SeaPeptide.com/aolinks.

You can also scan the QR code below with your smart phone's camera and it will bring you right to the page.

PART 1

DREAM

Part 1 is all about getting you in the right mindset for adventure, from why it works so well in motivating you to tips on keeping that motivation. So, with all of that, let's get started with why adventure works so well...

1

WHY ADVENTURE

On the morning of October 23rd, 2009, I was crying before I even opened my eyes. I rolled over, grabbed my meter from my nightstand, and tested my blood sugars. 458. And I was probably that high all night.

I could taste the ketones running through my veins and I swear my blood was as thick as syrup oozing its way around my body.

I got up and dragged myself to the kitchen to eat, but, of course, just the thought of food made me want to throw up. I didn't know what else to do, so I slid down the cupboard into a pile of tears right there on the kitchen floor.

I wish I could say that at that point in my life that was just one crappy day. We all have those. Those days when everything goes wrong and our sugars are just freakishly high.

But it wasn't. This was how every day of my life had become. My strength to test had vanished. I was so down about my numbers I avoided testing because it would be just one more bad number to look at. I hated having to deny myself my favorite foods every day. I found every excuse in the book to avoid my workout for the day.

At that point, I had been dealing with diabetes for twelve years. For the first few years, diabetes wasn't really that bad. Every time I would show up in Doc Wallace's office, he would give me a letter grade for my diabetes care for the last three months. I wanted to get a good report card from him, so I worked really hard. I always got A's, which, of course, I was really proud of. I knew I could beat a silly disease like diabetes.

But after a few years, getting a made-up grade from a doctor wasn't enough to keep me doing all the things I needed to do to stay healthy. And I got more and more lazy about diabetes.

I would put off testing till a little later, forget to put more test strips in my meter. I would let my pump run entirely out of insulin before I refilled it and, of course, I wasn't at home when that happened so I couldn't refill it right away. I would even forget to bring sugars with me wherever I went, which got me into some scary situations.

I wanted to take good care of my diabetes, I was just out of motivation.

A few minutes after I collapsed in the kitchen that morning, my husband came into the room. After a big hug, he told me to take the day off and figure this thing out. So I did.

I grabbed my laptop and headed for my favorite coffee shop, determined to dig myself out of this thousand-foot hole. I was smart. I could figure out some way to make all of this better.

If I could just try harder, make a different plan, write out some goals, I could push myself out of this mess by sheer force of will. Maybe I was doing so poorly because I wasn't trying hard enough, or I didn't care enough.

So I made an innovative plan and wrote countless goals. Things like test ten times a day. Go for a run every single day. Eat more salads for lunch.

But the moment I got back to real life, I forgot all of those goals. I failed within an hour of starting. And once again, I was at the bottom of an immense hole of diabetes, with no way to get out. I realized that making all those goals and lists would not be enough.

Luckily, during that day off, I ran across a group of people with diabetes that were super adventurous. They were running Ironman triathlons and hundred-mile races and climbing mountains. They inspired me to try my own hand at adventure.

When I was diagnosed with diabetes, my doctors laid out a list of things that I could no longer do. I couldn't drive a big rig, fly an airplane, or sail alone. I can remember sitting in the doctor's sterile office during my visit and swearing to myself that I would do just that. There was no way he was going to set limits on my life.

The time had come to make good on that promise.

At the very tip of Florida, there is this string of 1724 tiny islands that extend one hundred miles into the ocean like a giant fingernail at the end of the Florida finger. I decided I would sail from mainland Florida to the very end of that strip, to a place called Key West. And just to prove my doctor's wrong, I would do it alone.

I started planning right then for that adventure. And as I did, I found my motivation returning. My excitement and passion swelled up within me. I had energy to test my blood sugar and retest my basal rates. I started swimming again and exercising regularly. If I was going to sail safely, I had better be in great shape and be in superb control of my diabetes.

THE LONG ROAD

Diabetes is, for now, a lifelong disease. It is a monster that sits forever on our backs, constantly distracting and complicating our life. He demands blood and pain and tears. He craves restraint and self-control and moderation.

And he is never satisfied.

Never.

It would be easy to take care of diabetes if it were a month-long affliction. Even if it were just for a year. But an eighty- or ninety-year-long run is just too much.

We could try harder, push more, focus all of our attention on diabetes. We could forget about everything else going on in our lives to make our numbers perfect. We could spend every ounce of our energy on it. But in the end, we would end up with a life not worth living and it still wouldn't be enough.

Or we could do it differently. We could, instead, focus on something we love. Something that will make our hearts take flight. And something that will, as a by-product, better our diabetes care.

That something is adventure.

WHAT IS ADVENTURE?

Webster's dictionary defines adventure as an exciting or very unusual experience; a bold, usually risky undertaking; a hazardous action of uncertain outcome. When I think of diabetes adventure, it has to have three parts; travel, exercise, and enormity.

An adventure is something that brings us to new places. This world is vast, with so many amazing places to see. And I want to see them all. When we go to a new fresh place, it heightens our senses. We notice the small details. We pay attention to the experiences of new things.

The ocean smells saltier. The sun rises above the water instead of setting over it. These new sensations refresh us and bring us renewal.

Because we are using adventure to refresh our motivation to take care of our diabetes, exercise is also an integral part of adventure. Exercise reduces stress, challenges us in fresh ways, and makes our bodies more sensitive to the insulin we have.

It also combats some complications of diabetes by strengthening our cardiovascular systems and fighting heart disease. It gives us something to focus on as we train to take on such a big physical challenge.

Lastly, an adventure needs to be big enough to force us to take it seriously. If we are using adventure to change our lives and our relationships with diabetes, it has to be big enough to produce those changes.

But my big is not your big. You don't need to swim around an island or sail one hundred miles or run an ultra-marathon (which scares the crap out of me). It only needs to be big enough to challenge you, to cause you to reevaluate how you do things, and to inspire you to do more.

WHAT ADVENTURE DOES TO OUR BRAIN

The brain has different areas, used for different functions. There is a part for emotions, a part for math, a part for foreign languages, a part that tells you not to curse in church. Each part does something different.

There is even a part of the brain that fires up when we think about ourselves. Dr. Hal Hershfield did a study that looked at the parts of the brain that are active when we think about our present selves and our future selves and he found something unusual.

When we view ourselves now, we use the medial prefrontal cortex and the rostral anterior cingulate cortex. When we think about our future selves, we use the same parts of our brain we would when thinking about another person. Our Future Selves feel like someone else to us.

Hershfield's study illustrates that changing your behavior today to protect your Future Self forty years down the road is nearly impossible. Your brain sees that Future Self as someone completely distinct from your Present Self. So why deny yourself another cupcake if "that" person is the one to suffer? Why workout today, if "he" will be the one to pay later? There are no consequences to the Present You.

Diabetes has some short-term consequences—a low will ruin our day, a soaring high will make you feel crappy—but those long-term consequences, the enormous ones doctors try to threaten us with, they are decades away. And it is supremely difficult to always keep those in mind when the payoffs for splurging are immediate.

What you need to do is bring those long-term consequences into the present so your brain registers them as affecting the Present You. Adventuring does just that.

When I have an adventure on the books just a few months away, I make all of my decisions to ensure the success of that adventure. This cupcake doesn't have to destroy my kidneys in thirty years, it might add a few ounces to my body for my 100-mile paddle in three months. And the right decision is simple.

Another helping at dinner doesn't have to give me heart disease in forty years, it will make my training session tomorrow feel sluggish. No, thank you.

Getting up in the middle of the night to check my sugars doesn't have to cause nerve damage in fifty years, it will impede my recovery from a long paddle tonight. Get out that meter.

All of those decisions become simple. With consequences for the Present Me, I will make the right decision and take excellent care of myself. I have to. I have an adventure to get ready for.

SO LET'S GO...

Adventure will delight you with newfound motivation. It will challenge you physically as you train for it. It will counter complications with a stronger cardiovascular system. It will make far-off consequences more real. And it will provide you with amazing tales to share. So let's get going...

2

YOU ARE HERE

If you want to go anywhere, you need to get a grip on where you are right now. You can't make goals or plans if you don't know where you are starting from. So today it is time to take a long, hard look at where your diabetes adventure level is.

Because diabetes is such a long-term condition, it is very easy to grow complacent. A 200 blood sugar used to freak me out, but now sometimes I can ride the 300s for hours without flinching. A while ago I might have changed my insulin pen needle every day. Now it stays on the pen until it hurts. I plan on working out six days a week, but things always come up, and I only put in two on average.

And these minor changes go on without my notice. My care slips and I have no idea, usually, until something big happens.

The same thing happens in my adventurer life. At times I may find a mini-adventure to take on every day, seeking to make the most of every moment. Other times, I may let complacency take hold and never open my eyes to the possibilities.

I don't want to live like that. And I'm sure you don't either. The only way to overcome this is to live intentionally, and the first step is to get an accurate picture of what your reality is right now.

There are two parts to this inventory: the diabetes care side and the adventurous side. Take your time with each. Neither is more important. Look at what you are actually doing this week. Not what you think you are doing. Not what you know you should be doing, but what you are genuinely doing daily.

Just like the first step to losing weight is to track every morsel of food you put into your mouth and every bit of movement you make, the first step to your diabetes assessment is to track what you are really doing day-in and day-out.

So go grab a sheet of paper, pull up a note on your phone, find a worksheet or an app that will allow you to track your care for at least 3 days, or a week if you have the patience. What things should you track? Well, what things do you do to take care of your diabetes?

Record your shots, your pump settings, and your blood sugars. Download your pump and your CGM. Document what you eat, when you ate it, and why you ate it. Record every workout, intensity, and how you felt about it.

Once you have all that data documented, then take some time to evaluate it and get a good idea of the reality of your current level of care.

3

INSPIRATION BY MOVIE

One of my favorite ways to boost my excitement for a new venture is to watch an amazing movie about someone pursuing a huge goal. Sometimes all it takes is a few minutes. Other times I want to invest in an entire night.

So your assignment this week is to take a moment, sit back, and let the inspiration flow from the screen to your heart.

To get you started, here are some of my favorite doses of inspiration in movie form. You can find links to all of these at SeaPeptide.com/aolinks.

BILL CARLSON

Bill Carlson was the first type 1 diabetic to complete an Ironman in 1983. He was only twenty-three. ABC's Wide World of Sports did a segment on his race.

He was doing the race when an insulin pump was as big as a tape recorder. He had to insert his pump with a huge needle after the swim. It is crazy to think of what he accomplished with such ancient technology.

Twenty-five years later, he completed another Ironman and still regularly wins long-distance cycling races and has more energy than an eight-year-old high on Pixie Sticks.

DAVE CORNTHWAITE

Dave Cornthwaite left his semi-successful job to go on the adventure of a lifetime. He never came back. He has been completing his Expedition 1000 project, where he would take on twenty-five different 1000 mile journeys, and added a few other projects since. His videos explain how it all started and are a good place to get to know his adventure style, but you might also want to spend some time on his website to get more in-depth with all of his crazy adventures.

BLUE CRUSH

Blue Crush is still one of my favorite movies to watch to get me amped up for a new adventure. I don't know, maybe it comes from watching too many surf movies as a teenager, but any time I want to get jazzed up to train again, it is my go-to movie.

Anne Marie is an up-and-coming surf star in Hawaii who struggles with making rent and taking care of her little sister, all while trying to overcome her fear of wiping out at Pipe.

WITHOUT LIMITS

Without Limits is the story of Steve Prefontaine, a runner who made running the mile a performance worth watching. He had a view of what was possible and pushed hard to accomplish it.

Guided by an amazing coach, Bill Bowerman, Pre captured hearts with his wild running style and the audacity to challenge the established running governing body. He ran for the pure joy of running. He held all seven American records from 2,000 to 10,000 meters at one point.

And he lived life on his own terms. After watching this movie, I am often inspired to run again--and I HATE running.

CHASING MAVERICKS

Chasing Mavericks is the true story of Jay Moriarity, a young man who is saved from poverty and hardship when he finds surfing. Frosty Hesson, played by Gerard Butler, teaches him the discipline and hard work needed to safely take on an enormous wave like Mavericks. There are great training montages and much wisdom about respecting the power of the ocean and disciplining your body to do amazing things.

SEA PEPTIDE SWIMMERS

In 2014 the Sea Peptide Swimmers became the first-ever, all type 1 team to take on the 12.5-mile Swim Around Key West. Blair Ryan beautifully captured the event as well as the road trip we all took to get to the end of US 1 and all the fun that ensued.

Whatever movie you choose, let it inspire you to get amped up.

4

TIME TO GET YOUR FEET WET

Now that you have considered becoming a greater adventurer, it is time to get your feet wet with a mini-adventure. Your assignment this week is to choose one mini-adventure and complete it.

Use your body in a novel way and you will see how strong and capable you are. You might even meet some new adventurous people. You may find a new sport to love. Energy will abound as you try something new. It will fill you with a sense of accomplishment that will help as you plan your big adventure.

Here are thirteen ideas to get the juices flowing, but don't feel you have to pick one from this list. Feel free to improvise, as long as it is something new and fresh and just a bit out of the ordinary.

MINIADVENTURES

1. Try a new class. Many community centers or gyms have a huge list of classes. Find one you haven't done before and jump in.

2. Try a whole new sport. There are classes at Cross-fit gyms, gymnastic centers, parkour training centers, boxing gyms, and rock climbing gyms.

3. Sign up for a new team. Join a soccer team, a basketball league, a softball team.

4. What did you love to do as a kid? Go out and try it again. Did you love sprinting, go to a track and do a track workout. Did you love swimming? Get back out there. Double points if the water is under sixty degrees.

5. Take a train a few stops away and bike home.

6. Take a local safari to see some wildlife in your own area.

7. Climb the highest peak within fifty miles of your home.

8. What have you always seen people doing and thought to yourself, "Those people are so cool"? Was it hang-gliding? Or hot-air ballooning? Or playing beach volleyball in only a swimsuit? Go try that out. Maybe someone will look at you and think that you are the cool one now.

9. Go on a Work-to-Nature-to-Work adventure with some friends. Leave straight from work and head out to nature. Set up camp, have dinner, and sleep outdoors. Get up the next morning and head to work. You will have a clear head and probably a fresh dose of creativity at work the next day. What better way to use every moment to its fullest?

10. Sleep outdoors. Whether that's in a tent in the backyard, out in the wilderness, or under the stars on the beach, there is nothing like waking up to the sunrise and fresh air.

11. Watch the sunrise and the sunset on the same day. It doesn't count if you are doing both from your car or office building. Stand outside with a cup of coffee and take the time to watch the whole sunrise from the time before it peeks over the horizon to the time it is fully visible. Think about all the amazing things you want to get done for the day.

Then pause again at the opposite end of the day to bid farewell to our own personal star as it slips below the horizon. Think of at least three great things that happened that day or three things that you have in your life that you love.

12. Find the closest body of water and get in. Swim, wade, surf, dip a toe, paddle, or sail. Find some way to get in that water. You will return refreshed.

13. Share the joy of adventure and bring someone with you. Everything is a little funner (is that actually a word by now) with someone else by your side.

Which one will you choose? Go find some way of being active that is not your usual way, go a little outside of your comfort zone, and you will be greatly rewarded.

Then make sure you share your mini-adventure with the world by posting a pic online with the hashtag #AdventureOnBook and get your props for being a grand adventurer!

5

THE STORIES WE TELL OURSELVES

For five very long years, I was sick. And I don't mean diabetes. This was a whole new beast.

It started slowly. I began getting more tired than usual. I couldn't run for as long as usual. I started putting on weight and getting very short-tempered. Every aspect of my being changed, and not in a good way.

Five years later, I had a diagnosis, Hyperthyroidism, and a cure, nuking my thyroid with radioactive Iodine. We would kill my thyroid and then do a daily replacement of thyroid hormone, a much easier hormone to deal with than insulin. So technically, I was cured.

The only problem was, although my body had been cured—it would still take another two years to rebuild its strength and agility—my mind was still in sick-mode. The five years of being sick had taught me not to push too hard, to protect myself at every turn. Because if I went out and played a little too hard, I would be in bed for days trying to recover.

So I went from a girl who would jump at the chance to race anyone, anywhere, to a girl afraid to run even ten yards. I had to tell myself hundreds of times, "Don't push too hard. Don't go too fast." That mantra saved me from putting myself in the hospital. It allowed me to survive and still manage to stand upright.

But its time had passed. My thyroid was better, my strength was returning. That old spirited girl was not, however. I realized I needed to give my brain a little medicine, too.

GETTING IT BACK

Science tells us we become the stories we tell ourselves. If we experience something tragic, how we recount the experience in the days after, both to ourselves, and to others, will frame the way the story is recorded in our brain.

If we recount the story to ourselves as the most awful thing ever and that we were powerless to stop it, we store that memory wrapped in fear and horror. If instead, we log the story of our bravery in the face of danger, and all the things we did right to make it better, we wrap that story in pride and strength.

Knowing this, I had to change the story I was telling myself about my current physical condition. I had signed up to lead the Sea Peptide Swimmers in the 12.5-mile Swim Around Key West six months out, and I had to be in the right mindset if that was going to be a success.

I had been swimming for a couple of months since getting better, but still would not take up the challenge to race my husband in the pool. Before this whole thyroid thing, I would have been the one challenging him, time and time again, until I could beat him.

I went to my bathroom mirror and wrote on it, "You are no longer sick, You are a happy SWIMMER." Every morning, when I did my makeup, I would read that saying aloud. Every time I passed it to shower, I would read it. When I brushed my teeth at night, I read it.

And soon I believed it. I knew I was no longer sick; I WAS A SWIMMER. I believed it so much that just reminding myself that I was no longer sick, was too much of a reminder that I had been sick. So I erased the first part. But I left up for the next 18 weeks, "YOU

ARE A HAPPY SWIMMER," right next to my countdown of days until my race.

Saying that to myself daily had changed what I believed about myself. And that new belief changed my actions. I began behaving like the picture in my mind of how swimmers behave.

I chose fresh foods because I was a swimmer, and that's what swimmers do. I stood taller, because swimmers are proud. I stretched while watching TV at night because swimmers take care of their bodies.

The changed belief led to changed behavior.

So here is what I am proposing to you. Do you tell yourself you are a diabetic? Do you tell yourself there are certain things you can't do because you are a diabetic? Do you pull back, just a little, because you have diabetes?

Do you want to act like a good diabetic, or do you want to act like an athlete? Like an adventurer?

It is time to stop calling ourselves diabetics and start calling ourselves adventurers. So go to that place where you note your goals, or take a large piece of paper and tack it up next to your bed, or if you don't have a place, go to your bathroom mirror (chalk markers work amazingly, or a simple dry erase pen will do the trick. They both erase nicely.) and write it down. "I am no longer a diabetic, I am a..." Finish that sentence with whatever you want to see yourself as.

Then spend some time conjuring up your ideal image of an adventurer, or whatever strong noun you used. What kind of food decisions do they make? How do they view missing workouts? How hard do they push themselves while training? What types of social decisions do they make? Do they stay out all night, or treat sleep as a part of training, and not risk it? How do they see themselves? How do they hold themselves? How do they manage their diabetes so they can excel at their sport?

Every time you face a decision, make it like that athlete you pictured. I want to eat fruits and veggies and salads because that's what an elite athlete does. I'm going to choose water instead of soda because athletes need to hydrate. I am going to change my site every two days because athletes aren't lazy about their diabetes care. I am going to walk into that party with pride, knowing I just finished a two-hour paddle and got ready at the lagoon while everyone else just got ready at home.

Then, when you're done writing it down (and, yes, you actually need to write it down where you see it every day) and imagining what that athlete does, go share your new belief online using the hashtag #AdventureOnBook, and maybe throw a little love to the other adventurers who are going along with you in this journey.

PART 2

PLAN

Congratulations on making it through the first module. Hopefully, you have been able to dream about adventure and what yours might look like.

In this next section, I will bring you through planning your next adventure. Then, in the next two modules, we will discuss training for and executing your adventure.

Keep focusing on this and taking the time to really dig in and explore. You deserve this adventure and all the amazing benefits that come from this experience.

Don't forget to take the time to think about the reflection questions in your workbook and actually write down the answers to help solidify the concepts in your mind and make you more likely to follow through. Remember to enjoy the process and have some fun.

6

CHOSE YOUR OWN ADVENTURE

There are as many adventures as they are people. Finding the right one is critical to having a good time and staying safe. So where do you start in trying to find your adventure? It's time to analyze yourself.

When I finished writing and publishing Islands and Insulin, I knew it was time to take on another adventure. But I had nothing specific in mind. I had run triathlons since I got diabetes in 1996, and, although I loved them at first, my passion had run dry.

When I began triathlons, they were a bit of a rarity. It shocked people when I shared my racing stories with them. Lately, though, they had become commonplace. And I am not obsessed with the commonplace. I knew it was time to move on.

That, coupled with the fact that I was incredibly slow, spurred me on to try something new. I was a horrible runner and an average cyclist, but when it came to swimming, I was halfway decent. In my triathlons, I usually came out of the water in the top ten. By the time the bike was over, I was in the back half of the pack. And when I had finished running, they had already given the awards out and were packing up the race site. Triathlon was not my calling, but I could swim.

So I started looking for swim races. I had no real racing experience other than the quarter-mile swim in a triathlon, so I knew I wouldn't be doing any channel crossings. And I hate cold water, so it had to be some place warm. I needed to race during summer break so I wouldn't have to miss any school.

I plugged my requirements into a race calendar and came up with the Swim Around Key West. I had already been to Key West during my sail but didn't really feel like I had enough time to explore the city. And I wanted to bring Tony back to see the town that I had fallen in love with the first time around.

The problem was the race was 12.5 miles, which was a little too far for me alone. They had a relay category for three swimmers, which put my swim at 4.2 miles. Now all I had to do was find some equally crazy teammates, and I was ready.

WHAT EXCITES YOU?

Your adventure is out there, ready to be explored. All you have to do is narrow down the choices. The best way to do that is to ask very specific, yes-or-no or multiple-choice kinds of questions. If you ask too big of questions, you won't have any answers. So start small.

Do you like to be warm or cold? In the water, on the water, or on land? Are you a city-type, country-type, or somewhere in between?

Do you like roughing it, or would you prefer five-star everything? Do you like to be around a ton of people, just a few, or no one at all?

Are you comfortable running around only in a bathing suit for five days in a row or do you prefer more clothing on your adventures?

How long can you realistically take away from work, family, or friends? What is your budget? When can you leave? What kind of gear do you currently own, and what kind of budget do you have to purchase what you might need?

How much travel planning do you like to do? Should you pick

an organized race with a pre-set course, or do you want to choose your course and timeline?

Do you want to stay in your country or go to a faraway country? To a country with the same language as you or different? How safe should the place be?

How comfortable with this place is your spouse or parents? This shouldn't be a limiting factor, but if it is all the same to you, there is no need to freak them out. Save that for when it really will make a difference to your adventure.

What types of activities have you done in the past? What kinds of activities are you good at? What activities have you been yearning to try?

Where have you been wanting to go? Is there a way to tie in your adventure to that locale? I wanted to see North Carolina for years. The Stand Up Paddle Adventure in 2015 gave me a reason to go see it in an extraordinary way, from the water.

Do you have family or friends somewhere who could serve as a base of operations for your adventure?

What are your limitations? I cannot function on less than 6 hours of sleep. I absolutely cannot run long distances or do anything quickly. So I would be unwise to plan an adventure that requires these things. Go with your strengths and know your limitations.

Using your narrowed-down choices, go explore online. See what is out there that will match your criteria. Come up with a few ideas and run with them.

Find out how feasible, expensive, and realistic each one is. Then choose your favorite and throw the rest on the Someday-I-Will list for later on down the road.

Once you have decided on your next adventure, go share it with the world. Who knows, maybe someone there will want to join you or help you on your way...

7

DON'T ADVENTURE ALONE

Adventuring alone can get tiring. Nothing is more inspiring than sitting down with another person who understands diabetes and adventure and trading war stories or dreaming about amazing adventures you might take one day. There are so many amazing groups out there who can make that happen.

But with groups, you only get out what you put in, so get out of your comfort zone and be outgoing. You'll be surprised how quickly you bond with other people with diabetes. I have listed a few I am familiar with, but; I bet if there's not one listed in your area, it's still out there. You just need to go find it.

Remember links to all fo these groups can be found at Seapeptide. com/aolinks.

FABULOUS, ADVENTUROUS DIABETES GROUPS

Connected In Motion is a group of people with Type 1 diabetes who share a vision: to create a culture of support and engagement in diabetes self-management through peer-based experiential diabetes education, sport, and outdoor adventure. They are based out of Canada and bring like-minded individuals with Type 1 diabetes and their support networks together to hike, bike, paddle, camp, or just have a good time.

Riding on Insulin is a snowboard camp for the kids, but they also need volunteer counselors. What a great way to get involved and give back at the same time. They also are leading retreats and adventure camps as well.

College Diabetes Network, although not exclusively a group based on activity, college kids are bound to be active. Their mission is to empower and improve the lives of students living with Type 1 diabetes through peer support and access to information and resources. They are based in the US.

Team Blood Glucose brings together people with diabetes, or at risk of diabetes, to take part in all forms of cycling in a safe and friendly manner, providing peer support and firsthand knowledge to each other. They are based in the UK.

Diabetes & Exercise Alliance is a free, grassroots organization led by volunteers. They have chapters all over the US and the tools you can use to start your own chapter.

ALMOST AS GOOD AS IN-PERSON

Try to find a real-life, out in the wild group. But if you absolutely can't do that, join a Facebook group. There are plenty of great ones out there. Here are a few of my favorites.

SDT1D If you speak diabetonese, are a PWD, D-Mom, D-Dad, surrogate pancreas, Type 3, diabuddy, sugar buddy, have a sugar baby, celebrate diaversaries, ever experience glucoasters, flatlining, CDDs, cluster-beeps, have ever gone D-postal, are familiar with the terms basal, bolus, bat belt, poker, no-hitter, or SDD, then join us, and if you don't know what these terms mean, don't be afraid to ask!

Athletes with the 'Betes is a community of active people who manage diabetes while being active, fit, and engaged in regular exercise. Runners, swimmers, cyclists, triathletes, team sports such as soccer, basketball, baseball, and even your badminton enthusiasts, or bocce ball players!! If you are NOT a couch potato, let's call you an athlete, and if you are not comfortable with that description ... yet ... well, they will change that!!

Type 1 Diabetic Athletes is a group to discuss their workout routines and how it has benefited them. Topics of discussion will include programming, nutrition, and optimization of your health via diet and exercise. Feel free to post questions, information about T1D, athletic pursuits and accomplishments, etc.

Diabetes Ultra-Endurance Athletes is for type 1 and type 2 diabetic ultra-endurance athletes and similar #diabadasses. You know who you are. When the tips and tricks you get from your existing groups aren't anything you haven't already heard, when you're looking for the next epic thing and need to chat with someone who's already done it with one hand tied behind their back testing their sugar. Let's bust some myths!

You never have to do diabetes alone. So get out there are find some support whether it's in person or online, seek help. We all need it sometimes.

8

57 ADVENTURES TO SPUR YOU ON

Dreaming about your future adventures is one of the best parts of this process. It is the time when anything is possible. Before you have to rule out things because they are too time-consuming, too dangerous, or too expensive. Now is the time to let your brain run wild.

But in case your brain is having a hard time starting, I thought I'd give you a list of 57 adventures. Maybe one will be just what you are looking for. Maybe one will get you brainstorming in the right direction. Maybe a couple can go on your Someday-I-Will list for years down the road.

Look and see where you end up. Of course, you take on all adventures at your own risk. Please make sure you are over-prepared and super-trained for whatever event you choose.

1. Hike the Grand Canyon Rim-to-River-to-Rim in one day. Or, heck, go out and run it.

2. Run a race a distance longer than you ever have in a faraway land. If you've run a 5k, find a 10k or a half-marathon. If you've run a half-marathon, try a full.

3. Bike across America or whatever country you desire.

4. Swim around an island or from island to island.

5. Paddle 1200 miles around the entire state of Florida as part of the Everglades Challenge.

6. Float down the entire length of a river in some sort of contraption. Start where it starts and follow it to the end.

7. Hike the length of an entire mountain range like the 1100-mile Pacific Coast Trail.

8. Climb a mountain. Pick one near or far. Mellow or Everest. Make your mark and see the world from a unique vantage point.

9. Body surf the Wedge in Newport Beach, California, on a big day.

10. Kayak the Na Pali Coast in Hawaii.

11. Kiteboard the length of a state or country.

12. Ski Inn-to-Inn on the Catamount Trail, Vermont.

13. Surf every break of an entire region or state or country.

14. Sail an epic race like the Transpac or the Newport-Bermuda.

15. Flowboard every flowboarding house in your country.

16. Dive Djibouti on the Horn of Africa, one of the earth's greatest dive spots that nobody knows about. Try your hand at managing diabetes UNDERWATER!!!

17. Mountain bike the 142-mile Kokopelli Trail that leads from Fruita, Colorado, to Moab, Utah.

18. Raft down the Colorado River through the Grand Canyon.

19. Climb a volcano and look into it.

20. Canyoneer the Azores, a Portuguese archipelago in the Atlantic 900 miles off the European mainland.

21. Lead a survival weekend in a jungle, island, or mountain. Bring only what is necessary. Find the rest of what you need to survive Bear Grylls style.

22. Compete in a 4-, 24-, or 96+ hour adventure race.

23. Sea kayak from island to island in Fiji. Bring everything you need to survive in your kayak.

24. Sail around Cape Horn in Chile, or around a large island, or from England to the US.

25. Run the Ice Marathon in Alaska. It takes place in temperatures of -20°C, though the brutal wind chill whipping around your chops can make it feel another twenty degrees below that.

26. Swim from island to island in Sporades Isles, Greece, or the U.S. Virgin Islands.

27. Stand Up Paddle the entire length of the Intracoastal Waterway.

28. River raft a Class IV river.

29. Ride a horse the entire length of a state, carrying with you everything you need.

30. Follow a historical trail in the exact place people from long ago traveled. Find a covered Wagon and travel the length of the Oregon Trail.

31. Hike to see all the places where a favorite movie or TV show was filmed. Or to every place mentioned in your favorite book.

32. Hike Iceland in the near-eternal day in summer or during spring break when the island tends to get a bit crazy.

33. Dogsled across a barren wilderness.

34. Complete an Ironman triathlon in a faraway city.

35. Run a marathon in every state on the East Coast of America.

36. Take a train to the end of the line and ride your bike back home.

37. Run to every Lighthouse in a state.

38. Surf every wave pool on earth.

39. Hike Catalina Island in Southern California from tip to tip. This 25-mile hike gives amazing views of the mainland from the

top of each peak. It is about a three-day venture with some camping each night.

40. Rollerblade or use Cardiff Skate Company's new skates to cover one hundred miles of unfamiliar territory.

41. Geocache all the spots in an area.

42. Rock climb a huge mountain.

43. Surf the very best break on each continent.

44. Skateboard at one skate park in each state.

45. Ride a camel across a desert.

46. Hike the John Muir trail 211 miles from Yosemite to Mt. Whitney covering some of the most beautiful wilderness in the US.

47. Run from hotel to hotel carrying only a change of clothes and a credit card.

48. Do an "all boards" trip in Indo. Longboard, shortboard, stand up paddle, bodyboard, kiteboard, surfing canoe. Ride a wave on everything.

49. Sail around the world alone, with a friend, or on a team as part of the Volvo Ocean Race.

50. Explore the Son Doong cave in Vietnam. You can spend six days camping inside this enormous cave and hiking all around.

51. Build your own wooden boat and then sail it along the entire coastline of a state.

52. Try out volcano boarding, flying down the face of an active volcano on a reinforced plywood toboggan.

53. Downhill mountain bike at a ski resort in the summer.

54. Go freshwater cave diving in Mexico's Yucatan Peninsula.

55. Zorb across a city. A zorb is a transparent plastic ball you climb into and roll.

56. Coasteer a rocky coast. This requires you to traverse the intertidal zone of a rocky coast on foot or by swimming without any watercraft.

57. Combine three or more sports to cover a distance, like traversing the U.S. Virgin Islands by swimming, kayaking, biking, and running.

Hopefully, one of these adventures piqued your interest and got you thinking. Maybe a few did. Now go out and expand on that dream. Make the adventure especially yours. Find the details that make it attainable and safe. And then begin planning...

9

NAYSAYERS

You've got a spouse, parents, kids, friends, or a doctor. And living a life of adventure is not always a solo decision. It will affect those around you as you invest time and money into this process.

The good news is that adding adventure to your life will only increase your motivation to take care of your health and that will benefit everyone in your life. So I've anticipated some of the most common concerns you may hear from your loved ones about your new adventure—which are valid and worthy of consideration—and some equally valid arguments for why you must take on this adventure.

I've also included things you can say to help these people understand your actions and motivations. So, let's cruise through some of the most common questions you may hear.

COMMON CONCERN #1: This will be a huge investment of money.

What You Can Say: Although it does cost money to travel and buy gear, it gives me something that money can't buy. Adventure has lit a fire under me again. Because of my future adventure, I will take better care of my diabetes, which will save us money in the long run as I can avoid or delay complications which would cost ten times the money in medical bills, more prescriptions, and time lost from work because of sick days and leaves.

I will also choose an adventure that fits within our budget and lifestyle, and I will make a few sacrifices in the things I spend my money on now to make up the difference. This is really important to me. Are there things we can change in our budget to make this a reality? Can you get behind this?

COMMON CONCERN #2: What if this adventure takes all your time and there's none left for me/the family/your job?

What You Can Say: I admit, I am going to want to spend a ton of time planning and training for my adventure, and I will spend a few days traveling. But all of this training and planning will help me have more energy and passion for life.

I will be more fulfilled and happier because I am doing something for me, something that will make me healthier. And a happier me is more likely to go the extra mile with you/family/my job because I won't feel as burdened with the tasks of diabetes. Wouldn't you love to be around me when I am happier and more energetic? I know I would.

COMMON CONCERN #3: Adventure won't really make a difference in how you take care of your diabetes?

What You Can Say: Adventure pulled Erin Spineto out of a diabetic depression and has kept her from falling back in for over ten years, now. All of her teammates in her adventures demonstrated the same thing. They began focusing on maximizing their diabetes care to prepare for their adventure, and they have had renewed motivation and excitement to do it.

I am connecting with other people with diabetes, too, who are experiencing the same lift and who are encouraging me and supporting me. Those connections, alone, are enough to keep me jazzed about taking better care of my health. Isn't it worth a try to at least see if it will work for me? I would do anything to gain motivation and excitement about my diabetes again.

COMMON CONCERN #4: You've already invested in other systems, downloads, and programs that you stopped using after a few weeks.

What You Can Say: All of those required me to manufacture willpower. This is different. I don't have to force myself to do it. The excitement of an adventure is pulling me to do all of those things I have tried to push myself to do and failed.

Also, I am no longer doing things to make sure I avoid complications thirty years down the road. I make my choices based on what will make my adventure succeed this year. And it is much easier to follow through on things when the consequences are more quickly realized.

All of those other programs were things made up by other people and forced on me. My adventure is personal. I have chosen it to meet my needs and challenge me, not any other person on earth. And because I chose it, it is the perfect way to keep me motivated.

COMMON CONCERN #5: People with diabetes should not be too wild. Moderation is the key (This one is usually put forth by your doctor.)

What You Can Say: I am planning on _____ (type of adventure like swimming 4.2 miles). And it has been the greatest thing for my diabetes. I have tested more and going the extra mile to stay healthy. And I have been thinking about how to manage diabetes while I_____(type of activity like swimming) and I know you can help me.

How can I use my Dexcom and pump/insulin to make it as safe as possible? (You may want to ask a real-world problem you have come across, like how to avoid highs after a long workout, or how to get insulin coverage while swimming for hours without a pump on.) Are there things I may encounter in training and executing this adventure that you could help me make a plan for before I encounter them?

By presenting the benefits of adventure first, your doctor will see how important and useful it is. By asking him to help you solve problems and being specific, she may be more willing to come alongside you and help you solve them, instead of just saying you're crazy, although, most of my doctors call me crazy right before they help me solve problems.

Remember, doctors are smart people who love novel problems to solve in original ways. If you present them with a fresh problem, they will have a hard time not trying to solve it.

COMMON CONCERN #6: Isn't going on a grand adventure dangerous for a person with diabetes? I thought you weren't allowed to fly a plane or sail alone or do any strenuous or endurance sports.

What You Can Say: Exercise is one of the greatest tools I have in this fight. It makes my body more responsive to the insulin I use. It also helps me fight against some of the complications such as heart disease and high blood pressure. And if I have a reason to exercise, I will miss fewer sessions and push harder in each session.

Having diabetes today is a lot different from having diabetes twenty years ago. A lot of those warnings were from the medical knowledge of two decades ago. The technology we have today has made adventuring and endurance sports much safer.

My Dexcom Continuous Glucose Monitor will give me data continually and I can adjust my insulin pump basal rates or my long-acting insulin to prepare me for the exertion. I am gathering data and talking with my doctor to make those adjustments as I go along in my training.

I am reevaluating my nutrition before, during, and after all of my workouts. And I always carry a few sources of quick-acting sugar like Gu energy gels or juice.

I am planning my adventure safely, thinking of everything that may come up and how I might deal with it. Diabetes means that I have to do more planning, but it does not mean that I cannot go.

Is there something I can do while on my adventure to make you feel more comfortable, like checking in with you more frequently or walking you through my back-up plans for every possibility that might arise?

THEY REALLY DO LOVE YOU

Your loved ones are just concerned about you. The best thing you can do is listen to them and let them know you understand how scary this disease can be and how they may feel like they have less control than they would like.

Then reassure them you are doing an outstanding job and let them know what you need from them to make it easier on both of you.

You may find your friends and family aren't the only ones who will ask you these questions. At times, you may doubt yourself and bring up these "logical reasons" to talk yourself out of adventuring.

If you find yourself doing this, come back and read this list again and remember all the amazing things adventure can do for your life with diabetes.

10

FREAKING OUT

Hopefully, by now, you have a fairly good idea of what your adventure might be. You may have even started planning the specifics and started building a team. If not, keep thinking. Inspiration often strikes when we least expect it if we leave the idea on our minds throughout the day.

CREEPING DOUBT

There comes a point during the preparations for every one of my adventures, where I completely freak out. And it always happens at the time when the dream shifts into reality.

I usually start planning an adventure a year out. I pick something grand and exciting--probably something I had been dreaming about for years--and I spend the next few months adding details to those plans. Where I'll stay, who I'll go with, and what my training plan will look like.

The excitement builds as I flesh out that dream. My first training sessions go smoothly. Happiness overwhelms me as I buy new equipment and see new muscles appear on my body.

But then a strange thing happens as the weeks turn into months and the countdown to adventure written on my mirror gets smaller. The stark realization that this adventure thing is no longer just a dream hits me. It is real. And it is huge. And it is coming at me swiftly.

Doubt creeps in and tells me loudly that it is too far to go, that it is way too big of an adventure for me to complete. What was I thinking? It's impossible.

And what's worse, everyone knows about my trip. All of those people who told me I was crazy for doing something like this with diabetes were right. There is no way on earth that I will succeed.

FREAKING OUT IS GOOD

We have been working on the premise that adventure will provide us with the motivation we need to focus on our diabetes care. If the adventure is small, our motivation will be too. It will not force us to be at our best. It will become nothing more than a whisper in the back of our minds that we can so easily dismiss.

In order for this adventure to revolutionize our diabetes life, it has to call out to us. It has to be huge, right on that line of what is possible and what is not. This means, at some point in the process, we should doubt whether we can complete such a monumental task.

Doubt means that we have chosen something big enough to challenge us, something we're not one hundred percent sure we can finish. Something that will cause us to consider each decision we make as if it could be the one thing between finishing and failing. Doubt means we are on the right track.

YOUR DOUBT BASHING TOOLBOX

Even though doubt is a natural part of the adventuring experience, it does not mean that there is nothing you can do about it. First, of course, is to accept that it is a good sign that you have chosen the right adventure.

Second, is to get control of your thoughts. When they start to spiral out of control, finding fresh proof of how foolish you are to take on something this big, the easiest way to bring them back to reality is with a quick and easy saying. Some people call it a mantra, but I have never been big on the touchy-feely connotation of that.

For me, it's a quick and easy saying I can whip out when my thoughts begin to spiral. And the more you use it, the more powerful it becomes. It's a little like training a dog with a spray of water. Every time doubt presses in, you spray it with a cold dose of water, your mantra, to shock it into compliance.

In the beginning, you may have to repeat it over and over until your brain gets the hint. After a while, just the threat of using your mantra will shift your thoughts back to where they should be. Mine is simple and applicable to many situations, "You got this, Erin." That's right, I talk to myself using my own name. Researchers at the University of Michigan did a study that proved that when you talk to yourself, it is way more powerful if you use "you" and your own name instead of "me."

So, if University researchers say it's the way to talk to yourself, that's what I'm going to do. You can also use a mantra in the middle of training when you are struggling to finish. You pull out the mantra and it takes your mind out of the I-am-so-tired, I-have-to-stop rut.

Different things may work for each sport. When I am swimming or paddling, it is, "Ride the Glide," from the movie, Chasing Mavericks. (It helps that Gerard Butler used it in the movie.) When I am struggling while running, which is almost continually, I say "left foot in front of right," in pace with the sound of my footsteps.

Using phrases like these, over and over through the training phase will imbue them with power that you can tap into when you get to the dark time in your adventure, because, every adventure, if it is big enough, will have a few dark moments to contend with.

DOUBT ALWAYS PASSES

I find my big moment of doubt usually comes before my training starts to ramp up. I have a hard time with an hour-long workout, so I look at my training plan and realize that it is only a fraction of how long my workouts will be towards the end of my training plan. And just a sliver of the total distance I will have to cover on my actual adventure. The distance seems insurmountable.

After I wallow for a minute, I pull out my mantra and use it. I have to repeat it hundreds of times in the week between that difficult long training session and the one planned for the following week. But a strange thing happens that next week.

I usually have an amazing workout. Every moment is a joy. I push hard and finish strong. And I realize I can do this. I begin to trust in my training plan and in my own strength. The moment of doubt passes and I am back on track, highly motivated to maximize my diabetes and have the adventure of a lifetime.

So when doubt hits, and it surely will, thank it for reminding you that you have chosen the right adventure, and then fight it for all your worth.

PART 3
TRAIN

You're now halfway through. Hopefully, by now, you have a better idea why adventure is such a great tool for diabetes care and what adventure you might want to take on.

This module will focus on training so you might have a safe and comfortable adventure and avoid injuries. By the end of this module you should have a more complete knowledge of how to train, eat, and build new habits.

Remember to invest some time in the review questions because that is where the real work of adventure planning takes place. Now, let's get to it...

11

TRAINING STYLES

Rory Bosie is an unconventional ultra-marathoner. She wins most races, even placing in the middle of the top ten men. But in 2011, just four years after starting ultra-marathons, she could hardly walk up a flight of stairs without being winded.

The year before she had been picked up by the North Face Ultra team and started working with a Zimbabwean coach who increased the intensity and volume of her training. But with all of the focus and intensity, she began to get burned out.

The focused and intense training regimen that works for a majority of all the best ultramarathoners just was not working for her. Bosio reevaluated everything she was doing, and with the help of a long-time friend and sports-performance coach, changed the direction of her training.

She stopped running altogether and started skiing and hiking again. When she did resume running, she ran alone and without a watch, focusing on how running felt. She tapped into what works for her, which is really enjoying what she is doing. Her training plan is now based on making each of her workouts feel like a mini-adventure.

A training week for Bosio may consist of skiing, hiking, yoga, paddle-boarding, hula-hooping, riding her cruiser around town, or taking on a long run. She discovered that when she has a well-rounded schedule, it no longer feels like a workout, but like she is just out enjoying herself. She found what works for her and she is once again at the top of her game.

WHAT WORKS FOR YOU

Part of making a great training schedule is finding the perfect balance of stress and recovery. And finding what works for you. We are all built differently, both physically and psychologically.

What works perfectly for a pro triathlete might not work for you. What works for your spouse or best friend may mean the end of your athletic career. The best training plan is the one that takes into account your mental biases, your physical strengths, and your current lifestyle.

Finding out what works for you takes time and lots of experimentation. When I first started triathlons in college, I would train six days a week, sometimes even two workouts a day. But I would get fatigued and miss workouts, which would discourage me and I would get frustrated that I was not able to maintain an intense schedule.

As I got older, I started experimenting with different training plans. And what I found worked for me is a very untraditional plan. In training for my 4.2-mile leg of the Swim Around Key West in 2014, I put in one long swim on the weekends and one faster swim during the week focusing on speed or technique. I might throw in a slow run or long walk during the week also. But that was it.

And it worked for me. I found that I was fresh and strong for each long swim. I was no longer constantly fighting off the fatigue. And since my schedule was not overloaded, I could make every workout, which built my confidence. This training plan, or some version of it, is what I have stuck with since then.

Finding your perfect training plan takes a lot of experimentation and analysis. Think about your training in the past. What worked? What didn't? What made you love the sport? And what made you hate it? How easily do you get bored of doing the same thing over and over? Take what has worked in the past and see if it will work again for you.

But be open to changing things around. Even if something worked for you in the past doesn't mean that you won't have to continue to adapt it. You might have more or less stress in your life now due to work or kids or family. You might have to deal with new chronic medical conditions. You may live in a different climate. You may even be older. All of these factors will continue to change what makes a perfect training plan for you.

If you are regularly thinking about these stressors and analyzing your current and past plans, you will eventually come up with a plan that works for you. One that increases your desire to train and your ability to cover long distances.

WHAT WORKS FOR ALL OF US

Even though you need to adapt any training plan to your own personal style, there are some general principals that will make any training plan stronger. Every training plan should incorporate building, periodization, and technique.

BUILDING

A training plan should take you from the physical condition you are in at the beginning of training to where you want to be prepared for your adventure. But, just because you want to be able to run one hundred miles in two months, does not mean that there is a training plan that can do that. There are limits to how much you should build in any period of time.

The general principle is that any training plan should not increase in total volume (the total time or distance you cover in a week), or in the distance of your longest training session by more than 10% over the previous week. So, if you run ten miles total over the course of a week, the next week should be no more than eleven miles. If your long paddle was 100 minutes this week, it should be no more than 110 minutes next week.

Even though the human cardio system may be able to adapt to training quicker than this, the structures of the body may not adapt so quickly. It takes time for the muscles, ligaments, and tendons to become stronger. If you exceed this 10% rule, you risk injury, which will ruin your adventure or, at least, delay it.

With this 10% rule, it means that the amount of time that you can increase your training in any period of time is fixed. If you need to go from paddling sixty minutes to paddling two hundred forty minutes, it is going to take four to six months. Make sure you consider this when planning your adventure and give yourself enough time to build slowly and safely.

PERIODIZATION

The next principle of training is periodization. The human body cannot go at top speed forever. It needs periods of rest. So does your mind.

Periodization starts with the training week. Not every workout should be at 100% intensity. In fact, very few of them should be. During the week you should include long, slow workouts, high-intensity workouts, mellow, medium-distance workouts, and rest days.

The next area of periodization is the training block, which usually consists of three to five weeks. For the first weeks, workouts build in duration or intensity, with one week at the end of each block for a reduction of total volume.

This gives your body a chance to recover from the training stress. This is the week that your body builds itself back up to become stronger. Without it, you will never reap the full rewards of all your hard work.

The length of a training block will differ with each individual. What has worked for me is three weeks of training and one week of recovery. Newer athletes might want to start with two weeks of training and one of recovery. Experienced athletes may want to experiment with a longer training block.

Your entire year should also be periodized. The beginning of the training year should be focused on building an aerobic base and muscle strength. Then, slowly, training sessions get longer or more intense. At the end of your training year, which should coincide with your most important race or adventure of the year, you should be at peak form.

Then comes the most important part of the training year, the off-season. Each year, your body and mind need complete recovery. This part of your year, lasting from four to twelve weeks, gives your body a chance to completely repair any damage that the year has placed upon it. It is also a great time for your mind to recharge for the next year.

During this time, workouts will be unplanned and more spontaneous. They will be light and short. Many days will be spent on the couch. This is also a great time to focus on those areas in your life you may have neglected during the year; family, hobbies, or work.

Because of this change in activity levels, beware of rising blood sugars. This might be a good time to reevaluate your basal insulin levels and carb ratios. Checking in with a doctor at this time to help with that is also advisable.

TECHNIQUE

Technique in any sport is probably the most important aspect of training to avoid injuries. One workout a week, if not two, should be devoted to building your technique. If you have improper form, it places stress on joints and muscles that cannot withstand it. You will get injured. And that is the last thing any athlete wants.

Technique is learned slowly, through thousands of repetitions. Moving human limbs is a complex, multi-step process. To simplify it, the brain will put together strings of commands into one command. When you first learn to hit a baseball you have to think of every part of the process. Hands together, shift your weight to the front foot, twist your hips, swing your arms. Each time you make this movement your brain is putting together a sort of playlist. After a thousand or so repetitions, you no longer need to tell it to do each step, you just ask for the playlist and it plays it.

But if you have a bad song in the middle of that playlist, each time you play it, it will ruin the whole vibe, eventually causing you much pain. The key is to make sure that every song on your playlist is a good one.

Learn how to do your sport correctly. Find a coach, read good books, watch certified coaches go over drills on YouTube. Learn form early and practice it often. Then make sure your body knows the correct form.

This is done through form drills. These movements single out one particular part of your stroke or paddle or stride and overemphasize the correct way to perform each movement. You repeat them during your training session and then, during your regular workouts, try to recall those feelings and incorporate them into your workouts.

BUILDING A PLAN

Before you grab your new Stand Up Paddleboard and just go paddle for the first time, or grab whatever gear you need and do your sport, take the time to build a comprehensive training plan.

Accurately assess your current level of fitness and the level of fitness it will take to complete your adventure comfortably. Look at the training plans that have been developed by respected coaches in your sport. Then adapt the best one to your training style.

Taking the time to think about your training will ensure that you are ready to adventure. Any adventure will be much more enjoyable when you are physically ready to conquer it.

12

FINESING NEW HABITS

By now you have been thinking about your new adventure. Soon, if you haven't already, you will need to build some new habits in order to get ready for it. But you don't have to walk uphill both ways to make it happen.

There has been a lot of research done in brain science lately. Scientists are discovering that new habits are not built by brute force of strong will power. There are much more effective and easier ways to build new habits.

Below are a few of my favorites. Most of them I have come across on the website of James Clear of Stanford University who specializes in habits and routines. If you have a few moments, he has a great website and newsletter that will help make your habit building easier and more successful.

SYSTEMS NOT GOALS

When trying to build a new habit it is far more important to focus on the system you will use to get there instead of the actual goal. For example, your goal might be to finish a marathon. The system is the training that you will do every day to get there.

If you focus only on your goal and ignore your system, you may or may not get there. But if you focus only on your system, you will make significant progress, whether or not you think about your goal. If all you do is think about the 26.2 miles you have to cover, you may or may not actually train. But, if you focus on your daily run, every day, you will certainly be ready come race morning.

There are two benefits of focusing on the system, not the goal. Focusing on a goal denies your current happiness. It brings you into the mindset of, "Only when I can run a marathon, will I be happy." Focusing on the system allows you to enjoy the process and each mini-success.

Each time you complete a training run, you will feel successful and happy. Your happiness during the run will also increase because of the sense of pride that you will have in completing one more step.

Focusing on the system and not the goal will also bring your new habit beyond the marathon and propel you to your next goal. Achieving a goal, whether it is finishing a marathon or losing ten pounds, often brings on a period where people stop their new habit.

They have finished their goal, so there is no need to keep up with the new habit. Focusing on the system will propel you forward even when you have finished your goal so that the new habit will become a permanent one.

Focusing on the system also takes the sense of failure out of not making your goal. If you have the worst day of your life and have to pull out of your adventure, because you focused on the system not the goal, you still have succeeded. You have built a new habit that you can take with you.

MAKE THE RIGHT CHOICE THE EASY CHOICE

Now that you are focusing on the system, let's build a brilliant system, one that is easy and plays on what your brain naturally tends to do. The first way to do that is to make the right choice, the easy choice.

Most times our brains are overloaded and tired. They don't want to make difficult choices. It is really hard to motivate yourself to make it to the gym after a long day at work. They don't want to choose water over diet soda, or grab a bowl of veggies for a snack.

But they do want to do whatever is easiest. So make the right choice, the easiest choice. Make sure the diet soda is difficult to obtain. Don't stock it at home, or put it in the cupboard, so that to enjoy it you have to get a glass and fill it with ice first. Make water easy. Fill a water bottle each morning and keep it with you.

Figure out what would make your good choice easier to make. Do the work beforehand, like cutting up veggies each Sunday and pre-filling small containers with dip so you can just grab them and go. And make the wrong choice really difficult to make. Hide the cookies on the top shelf at the back of the cupboard.

CUE YOUR NEW HABIT WITH LOCATION

Most of us really want to start new, healthy habits. When we decide to start something new, we start out strong. For the first few days, we complete our habit without fail. But then life gets in the way and we get busy and, most of the time, we just forget to do it.

So let's make it really difficult to forget. The way to do this is to set up a cue to remind yourself. Your cue can come from a location, a time, another habit, or another person.

Our environment plays a huge role in the things we choose to do. Using this to our advantage is crucial. This can be as simple as placing foods we want to eat in the front of the fridge and on the counter where we will see them. You can also use location to place visual reminders of your habit.

My bathroom mirror is covered with writing. I have a grid where I write out my monthly goals in each of the four areas of my life; family, business, health, and personal. Each morning, as I get ready, I look over each goal and make a specific plan of how I am going to make progress in each area that day. Without it being thrown in my face each morning, I would go weeks without thinking about these things.

Place the tools of your new habit in plain sight. Put your dumbbell next to your desk to remind you to punch out a few bicep curls each day. Place your running clothes on your nightstand at night so they are the first things you see when you wake up. Put your gym bag in front of the door so you have to step over it to leave. Make it nearly impossible not to see the things you need to complete your habit.

CUE WITH TIME

Another great cue is to tie in your new habit with a particular time. That can be always going for a long workout on a particular day of the week. I have a really hard time remembering to get in my workouts in during the week.

Something always pops up, and then one thing leads to another, and soon it is eight at night and way too late to get a paddle in. So I have tied my long paddle to Sunday. Not a Sunday goes by that I don't know Sunday=Paddleday.

Another great way to cue a new habit is to tie it in with something you already do every day. Make it a part of your morning routine. Or do something the moment you get home from work. Do it at 7 each night.

When my kids were young, we put them to bed each night at 6:45. As soon as we finished the bedtime routine, my husband would fire up P90x and we would complete our workout for the day. We knew as soon as those kids were in bed; we were working out. We never forgot a day.

CUE WITH ANOTHER PERSON

Working through P90x each night was also so much easier because I did it with my husband. If I had a particularly hard day, I might have been tempted to skip a workout. But knowing that he was there, already dressed and warming up, made it mandatory that I show up.

And usually within ten minutes of working out, I was glad I did. The tired feeling that tempts us to skip workouts is usually banished within moments of starting. That feeling really should be a sign that we need a workout more than ever.

Sticking to a new habit becomes so much easier when we do it with another person to hold us accountable when we are feeling low. We also have the chance to help that person when they are feeling low, which actually increases our confidence in our abilities and drives us to continue with our habit.

REWARDS

If we want our brain to like participating in a new habit, we need to begin to associate positive feelings with the activity. That can be done with rewards.

The simplest way of doing this is to develop a system to reward yourself after a number of successful activities. One solid week of making every workout gets you a new pair of socks. Or each run earns you one dollar in the new workout outfit jar. Making the reward related to the new habit you want to build will also reinforce those positive feelings, whether it's new equipment or a trip where you can test your skills.

Another reward system is called "temptation bundling." This is the one I have used to get me on the treadmill in the garage at 5:30 each morning for months at a time. It involves something you really like to do and something you know is good for you, but you have a hard time doing.

For me, I enjoy watching—and I hate to admit this publicly—I like watching my DVD collection of Dawson's Creek. So I made myself a promise that I would only watch it while I'm on the treadmill. If I want to find out what happens in the next episode, I will have to fire up the treadmill for another forty-two minute run.

This way I feel good about my run and I get to do something I really like. Plus, it means I don't watch Dawson's Creek on the living room TV, which is a huge plus for my husband who can't stand to be in the same room when the show is on.

The last reward system was proposed by Jerry Seinfeld. The system he used to become such a great comic was to write jokes every day. He would take a huge calendar and, for every day he wrote for an hour, he would mark a big red X over the day. After a few days, it made a chain. And he would do everything he could to not break the chain.

You don't have to use a calendar. You could use a chain of

paperclips, or paper strips, like the chains we used to make in grade school for Christmas decorations. For each day you complete your habit, you put a link on the chain. If you miss a day, the whole chain comes down.

Once that chain gets long enough, there is no way that you would want to break the chain. Putting it somewhere visible daily will also make it becomes a great reminder of how much hard work you have put into your new habit.

MAKE IT HAPPEN

So, go beyond just choosing your goal. Be specific about how you plan to get there and then focus on the process. And set up your life to ensure success. Make every step of the process a little easier and you will be on your way to a much more disciplined life.

13

INSPIRATION BY BOOK

It's time for another round of inspiration. This time it's coming from books. Anytime I am stuck inside in the winter, or bogged down by too many responsibilities and I just don't have the time to go out on a weeklong adventure, I can always find time to squeeze in a little adventure reading.

My reading tends towards sailing adventures, but I stray from time to time. Below is a list of my favorite adventure books and some that I have on my to-read list.

Sailing Alone Around the World In 1898, Captain Joshua Slocum was the first man to circle the globe alone on a 34-foot sailboat. In a little over three years, he did what many experts said was impossible. He was chased by pirates, met a few interesting people, and went a little crazy. It is a classic story of a man doing what many told him he could not.

A Pirate Looks at Fifty by Jimmy Buffett I am a big fan of Jimmy Buffett's music and business prowess, much more than his writing style. Although Jimmy Buffett is a much better performer than he is a writer, his adventures are fun. It was a fast read and one of the few books I've read where there were no death-defying survivals, just some good old travel fun.

The Longest Way Home: One Man's Quest for the Courage to Settle Down by Andrew McCarthyis the travel adventure story of the cool guy in Pretty in Pink trying to grow up for real. McCarthy may be a quintessential actor of the 80s, but I think his calling really should have been as an author. His writing is lovely and quick. And his adventures lead him to a fuller understanding of himself and his most prized relationship, which is what all adventure should do.

Close to the Wind by Pete GossandGodforsaken Sea by Derek Lundyboth tell the same story of the 1996-1997 Vende Globe, now the Volvo Ocean Race, a four-month sailboat race around the world via the Southern Ocean that went all wrong. Pete Goss heard a Mayday call from a fellow competitor. Without hesitating, he turned his boat around to sail back into the Antarctic hurricane he had just sailed through, barely surviving, to save fellow competitor, Ralph Dinelli, thus ending his own race.

The Art of Non-Conformity by Chris Guillebeau, although not an adventure book per se, is a book that challenges you to look at your life and question the givens you have accepted since birth. It also gives you the tools to live differently.

Islands and Insulin: A Diabetic Sailor's Memoir by me. (Of course, I had to add this one.) It's not as big of an adventure as the Vende Globe guys, or Captain Joshua Slocum, but it does have the diabetes spin. If you haven't read it already, it is the story of my 100-mile solo sail in the Florida Keys to prove to doctors that diabetes cannot put constraints on my life.

So fire up that Kindle or go on Amazon and order away. Or you could be really adventurous and go into a real bookstore. Your vicarious adventure awaits.

14

NUTRITION 101

When I was diagnosed in 1996, the doctor gave me a meal plan that laid out what types of foods I was to eat at each meal and snack. He also gave me my dosing schedule of Regular and NPH insulin that would not change from day to day. Every day had to be the same foods at the same time, along with the same insulin regimen.

I tried to stick to the plan, but the plan didn't match my life. The college life-style was always changing. Thursday afternoons, I worked with a youth group and we served them ice cream and candy at 2 p.m. Tuesday nights, after Bible Study all of my friends would go out to eat at ten at night.

No doctor was going to build me a meal plan that has an enormous meal at 10 at night. So, I learned quickly to make my own. I figured out how big of a bolus I would need and gave myself the extra insulin before my meal. It wasn't long before I realized shots weren't going to match my way of thinking.

Nine months after being diagnosed, I got my fist insulin pump. And after nine months of eating on schedule, I was free. It was that day that I actually felt hungry for the first time in a year. I no longer had to eat because it was time. I could now eat when I was hungry.

And I took full advantage of that fact. I ate whenever and whatever I wanted. All I had to do was count the carbs and give myself the right amount of insulin. By the time my next blood test came around, most of the time, I was back in the "good" range.

It wasn't until I started with my Dexcom CGM, that I figured out that, even though I could match insulin to my foods and get back in the good range in a few hours, not all foods affected me the same way.

Even though I can calculate insulin for a candy bar, I am going to get a blood sugar spike from it in the two-hour window after I eat it. If I have a Kachava, my blood sugars will remain completely stable during that two-hour window.

As people with diabetes, we have to focus so much of our attention on eating to balance our blood sugars we forget that food affects other areas of our physical life. That candy bar is going to leave me hungry about an hour after I eat it. Kachava will power me through a two-hour workout.

The foods we choose will affect not only our blood sugars, but our ability to adventure and our overall health. Just because we have diabetes, doesn't mean that we get to neglect these other areas when it comes to food choices.

CARBS TO FUEL EXERCISE

One of the biggest mistakes I see beginning diabetic adventurers make is the view that the only time we fuel during a workout is when we are low. Simple sugars go on that list of foods we are only "allowed" to eat when we are low.

But every athlete needs a source of sugar when they are exercising for over ninety minutes. The challenge for us is to figure out how to balance insulin with those extra carbs.

Some people will reduce their basal insulin to help with the exercise lows and then bolus for their nutrition during a workout. Some people will keep their basal insulin the same (especially for those on Multiple Daily Injections, or MDI) and then eat a regular amount of carbs at regular intervals, depending on the intensity and duration of their workouts. During a really tough workout, someone might even keep their basal rate the same and bolus for the extra carbs.

The key here is to figure out, with your doctor if needed, what system works for you for each sport. But don't avoid the extra carbs during long workouts. It is likely to make you sluggish and weak and hit the wall even sooner.

EAT REAL FOODS

If we have our insulin regimen dialed in, we can technically, just as every other person, eat whatever we want. But even though we can without the diabetes police arresting us, does not mean that we should.

The typical American diet is one that is taking a toll on our population. The foods we consider normal are not in the least bit healthy. They won't make us stronger. They won't give us more energy. They won't do anything, but fill our bellies for the moment and drive us to eat more garbage.

There are plenty of fad diets and people who will tell you that the only way to eat is exactly as they do. There are wackos on social media who will tell you only to drink water with hot peppers and guava juice for three weeks and it will fix all of your problems. Please avoid these guys at all costs.

Focus instead on some solid, biological, nutritional facts. We need nutrients and calories. Our bodies take in fat, carbohydrates, and proteins, break them down to rebuild all the structures in our bodies with those parts. And with soil health diminishing, reducing the quality of foods, we also need to take in vitamins and minerals to do the same thing.

For your body to run at its peak, focus on foods that are real. That means they look very similar to what they looked like when they were pulled out of the ground. The less that people and machines mess with your food, the more your body will like it. These foods are filled with vitamins and minerals and fill you up so you naturally eat the right amount.

One way to see how much your food has been changed, destroyed and rebuilt with artificial parts is to check how many ingredients it has and if you can read those ingredients. The fewer, the better. "Potatoes, oil, salt" would be a decent list for a potato chip.

"Enriched corn meal (corn meal, ferrous sulfate, niacin, thiamin mononitrate, riboflavin, and folic acid), vegetable oil (contains one or more of the following: corn, soybean, or sunflower oil), salt, maltodextrin, sugar, monosodium glutamate, autolyzed yeast extract, citric acid, artificial color (including red 40 lake, yellow 6 lake, yellow 6, yellow 5), corn syrup solids, partially hydrogenated soybean and cottonseed oil, hydrolyzed soy protein, cheddar cheese (cultured milk, salt, enzymes), whey, onion powder, whey protein concentrate, corn syrup solids, natural flavor, buttermilk solids, garlic powder, disodium phosphate, sodium diacetate, sodium caseinate, lactic acid, disodium inosinate, disodium guanylate, nonfat milk solids, sodium citrate, and carrageenan,"

clearly means a lot had to be done to that food before it got to your plate.

Try to eat foods that don't even need an ingredient list, like apples, carrots, lettuce, and zucchini. And the more cooking you can do at home, instead of eating out, the cleaner your diet will be.

FOODS TO FIGHT COMPLICATIONS WE'RE AT RISK FOR

Diabetes will exact a toll from our bodies. We are already at a higher risk for cardiovascular disease and strokes. We have extra stress put on our bodies from fluctuating blood sugar levels. Let's not add any more stress.

Foods that are artificial and devoid of nutrients put a huge stress on our bodies as they have to break down and process them. High-fat and sugary foods will hurt our cardiovascular system in the same way as our diabetes will.

We can only do so much to avoid the damage from diabetes, but we are in full control of the types of foods we make our body digest and eliminate. Let's choose foods that will reduce the extra inflammation from blood sugar levels, things like fresh fruits and vegetables, seeds, beans and nuts.

These foods have nutrients that calm the inflammation and make our cardio system stronger, not weaker. They will fight off complications just like good blood sugar control will. Our foods can become another weapon in our arsenal in the fight against complications.

MAKE CHANGES SLOWLY SO THEY STICK

If you decide to make huge changes in the foods you choose to power your body, it is usually easiest to overhaul one meal at a time. So start with breakfast. Pick three of four breakfast options that are healthy and appetizing and switch them out for two to four weeks. The success that you feel from achieving a small goal will drive you on through the next phases.

Once you have settled in to the new normal, switch up lunch. Give yourself about two to four weeks to adapt to the change before moving on to the next one. Then go on to switch out all of your meals and snacks.

And leave yourself a little wiggle room for an occasional splurge. Occasional, meaning every once in a while, not every meal. Find a rate that you can live with. My splurges are usually when someone else is cooking, so I can enjoy the moment without letting food issues interrupt a good time.

And then, of course, when I want to spend a few quality moments with one of my kids and we head off to the local yogurt shop.

We are all creatures of habit. Once we find the foods we like, we pretty much choose from the same few foods at each meal. We have the same foods on our grocery list week after week. And we do this so we don't become overwhelmed by all the choices we have to make.

Once you have settled in to the new routine, it won't be any harder on you to make great food choices. You just need to retrain your choices for a little bit, and then they will be the new normal for you and you won't have to give it an extra minute of thought.

FIND A LOW STRESS TIME TO MAKE THE CHANGES

For the time period when you are retraining your brain, you will have to focus a little more energy on changing your systems. It will take a little bit of will power to break old habits and form new ones. Make sure you are using the strategies we talked about on Day 12 to build these new habits.

And chose a time in your life when stress is naturally lower. Right before the holidays is probably not the best time to start a new routine. There will be far too many changes in routine with all the extra parties and events, and overall, stress is higher during the holidays.

My favorite time to do a diet overhaul is during summer. I am off of teaching for twelve weeks and all the summer produce looks so good. I just want to be in the sun all day and eat fresh fruits and salads.

Another great time is right before school starts in the fall. We all start new routines for the school year and I love to take a few days to find new recipes that the family will like so that, when the stress of the school year is in full swing, I already have my go-to recipes when I don't have the extra energy to think about it.

CHOOSE HEALTH

Choose your foods for your optimal health, not just your optimal blood sugars. Luckily the foods that are good for your health are also excellent for blood sugar management. Set yourself up for a successful change by choosing the right time and take it slowly. And then congratulate yourself in a big way when you succeed.

15

THE AGGREGATION OF MARGINAL GAINS

Cycling on the Tour de France is a grueling life of non-stop torture. The race itself is a twenty-one-day race, covering 2,664 kilometers that take the riders around the country of France.

And although the race is long, the preparation for the race is exhausting. Riders will put in over 1,000 km a week for nearly fifty weeks a year. And to make it to the level of the top riders, they will need to do it for several years.

The race also requires riders to perfect different specialties. They will need to be strong climbers for the mountain stages, have a top-speed engine for the time-trial days and for sprinting to the finish line each day, and overall endurance for the staggering miles they will cover in this incredible race. Only the most balanced riders will come out on top.

Because it is so grueling, the Tour is a prestigious race. Countries will spend an enormous amount of time and energy trying to win. In 2010, the British Cycling team was failing in this pursuit. They had never won a Tour de France.

When Sir David Brailsforde became the team's General Director in 2010, he was tasked with developing a winning team within five years. He did it within three. That same year he took the British cycling team to the Olympics and claimed over 70% of the medals in cycling. And he did it all with the concept of the Aggregation of Marginal Gains.

Brailsforde didn't walk into this job and tell the cyclists to train harder, as if they somehow were dogging it. These were professional cyclist who put everything they had it their training. Telling them to do better was not going to change their losing streak.

Making these men into champions was going to take a whole new approach. Brailsforde knew he would need to improve on every aspect of his athlete's lives and if he could do that by just one percent, all of those one percents would add up to an amazing change.

He began by looking at the usual things, like the athletes' training and racing schedule. He then looked for one percent improvements in how they recovered from workouts. He analyzed their diets on and off the racecourse and made slight tweaks.

Brailsforde looked at the type of pillow that would increase the quality of sleep. He even brought in experts to teach the team how to properly wash their hands so they could reduce illness and the time and energy it takes away from training.

All of those one percents added up to a winning team.

THE ONE PERCENT OF DIABETES

The Tour is a lot like diabetes. It is a never-ending endurance race that requires us to balance so many things. We have coaches who tell us to just try harder, as if we aren't already trying. But the same philosophy that took Britain to number one on the Tour can take us to number one in our diabetes care.

What if we gave one percent more in every aspect of our diabetes care? What if we tested one percent more often, or one percent sooner? What if we ate one percent better, avoided one percent more desserts? What if we bolused one percent sooner or corrected at a level one percent lower? What if we worked out with one percent more intensity or skipped one percent fewer workouts?

What would be the result if we did all of these one percents? Giving one percent more effort in every area will give us a huge difference when it comes time to get those A1c's down or when it comes to putting off the complications we are all trying so hard to avoid.

The magic of the One Percent Better, or the Aggregation of Marginal Gains, is that the changes are totally attainable. Anyone can squeeze just one percent more out of themselves. It is not a number that is so big that it scares us into avoidance. One percent is doable in almost any situation. But the one percents in every area will build upon each other.

So the next time you feel a little high and you are considering putting off testing until your TV show is over, think about One Percent Better, push pause and go test. Give yourself a bolus when you start eating your meal instead of twenty minutes after you have finished. Push yourself through one more sprint or rep at the gym.

Over the next thirty years of your diabetes care, think about how all of those one percents, day after day, will add up. If you were to invest one dollar a day for the next thirty years you would have over ten thousand dollars. How much more health will you have then, if you did everything just One Percent Better?

PART 4
EXECUTE

So you've made it through the first three parts. By now, hopefully, you have a good idea of why adventure is critical to a healthy life, what adventure you might choose, and how you are going to go about preparing for it. Now it is time to execute this plan...

16

THE SHOULDERS OF GIANTS

To help you along the way, I thought I'd share a few pieces of wisdom that I've run across in the past few years. They said it better than I ever could. If you find one in particular speaks to you, put it up where you can see it and let it motivate you to do your best.

At a certain point, it is time to move beyond dreaming and planning, and to start doing.

"Do, or do not. There is no try." —Yoda, Star Wars

"The secret of getting ahead is getting started." —Mark Twain

"The way to get started is to quit talking and begin doing." —Walt Disney

"If you want to be comfortable, don't try to live your dreams." —Emily Trinkaus

"You don't have to be great to get started, but you have to get started to be great." --Les Brown

"If you really want to do something, you'll find a way. If you don't, you'll find an excuse." —Jim Rohn

"A goal is just a wish with a plan." —Antoine de Saint-Exupery

"A year from now you may have wished you started today." —Karen Lamp

Adventure will show us what we are made of.
"The harder the conflict, the more glorious the triumph." —Thomas Paine

"One finds limits by pushing them."—Herbert Simon

"We must all suffer one of two things: The pain of discipline or the pain of regret." —Jim Rohn

"Let your dreams be bigger than your fears, your actions louder than your words, and your faith stronger than your feelings." —Unknown

My favorites from Steve Prefontaine, one of the best American runners ever, and his coach Bill Bowerman. Together, they made running more than just running. I have learned much about life from reading about these two men.
"To give anything less than your best is to sacrifice the gift." —Steve Prefontaine

"A lot of people run a race to see who is fastest. I run to see who has the most guts, who can punish himself into exhausting pace, and then at the end, punish himself even more." —Steve Prefontaine

"Somebody may beat me, but they are going to have to bleed to do it." —Steve Prefontaine

"The best pace is a suicide pace, and today looks like a good day to die." —Steve Prefontaine

"If you have a body, you are an athlete." —Bill Bowerman

"The real purpose of running, is not to win a race, it is to test the limits of the human heart." —Bill Bowerman

"There's no such thing as bad weather, just soft people." — Bill Bowerman

"Men of Oregon, I invite you to become students of your events. Running, one might say, is basically an absurd past-time upon which to be exhausting ourselves. But if you can find meaning, in the kind of running you have to do to stay on this team, chances are you will be able to find meaning in another absurd past-time: life." —Bill Bowerman

"Citius. Altius. Fortius. It means Faster. Higher. Stronger. It's been the motto for the Olympics for the last 2500 years. But it doesn't mean faster, higher and stronger than who you are competing against. Just Faster. Higher. Stronger. —Bill Bowerman

Adventure always brings with it risk. I will always be glad I took the risk.

"I am thankful for my struggle because without it I would never have stumbled on my strength." —Alex Elle

"Do one thing everyday that scares you." —Eleanor Roosevelt

"If it doesn't work out, there'll never be any doubt, that the pleasure was worth all the pain." —Jimmy Buffett

"You can never cross the ocean unless you have the courage to lose sight of the shore." —Christopher Columbus

"Inaction breeds doubt and fear. Action breeds confidence and courage. If you want to conquer fear, do not sit at home and think about it. Go out and get busy." —Dale Carnegie

"One of the inescapable encumbrances of leading an interesting

life is that there have to be moments when you almost lose it."
--Jimmy Buffett, A Pirate Looks at Fifty

And if it all goes bad, just ask...

"What would Pop-eye do in a tight spot like this?" — Jimmy Buffett, Take It Back

Do you have other amazing quotes that have served to inspire and motivate you in the past? Throw it up on Instagram and tag @erinspineto.

17

PLAN B, C, D, E...

When I was preparing for my solo sail, I found only one way to overcome all the excitement and put myself to sleep. I would visualize the worst possible thing that could happen during my adventure.

The weather got stormy. So dark and stormy that I was in danger of capsizing. The waves crashed over the deck, soaking everything I had onboard and filling up the cabin below.

The land was nowhere to be seen. My charts had been ripped out of my hands by the wind. And my GPS ran out of batteries. And then it happened. Azia tips. The weight of the thousands of gallons down below pulls her over and keeps her that way.

Soon the waterline sweeps up my body and then over my head. I have to unclip my lifeline and thrust my body towards the heavily churning surface. When I wipe the salt water from my eyes I can see *Azia*, now twenty feet from me, struggling to right herself, but it is a lost cause. I am on my own now.

Time to think. What would I do if that was what happened?

With no land in sight, my only source of direction is the driving waves. I noticed earlier they were sweeping at an angle towards land.

If I can follow them along, I might end up washed up on one of the uninhabited mangrove islands.

But, with the current running and the waves pushing me, I might miss land at the end of Key West and be dragged out to sea. Try again.

How about a thirty-degree angle to the direction of the waves? It may mean more swimming, but I have a better chance of hitting land. Last I knew, I was a half-mile from shore. But I could have been dragged away during the storm.

So, with the current and new distance, maybe a two-mile swim. I think I should probably increase the distance of my long training swims to make sure I can swim at least three miles before I take off. And I should make sure I have a life vest I can still swim with.

If I do hit land, it will be dark and full of shrubs. I can try to find shelter and weather the storm before finding a way to civilization, but all of my insulin supplies are at the bottom of the ocean, my pump is now water-logged and I have no way of testing.

Under this stress, I can probably only survive for 24-48 hours without any insulin and those will be a miserable 48 hours. I must get to civilization.

I've memorized the map of the keys. Most of the outside keys in the Lower Keys are mangrove. I have to follow them to the gulf side and then I can find some people. I may have to cross water at some point, but it is shallow and protected from the larger waves of the Atlantic Ocean.

Once on an inhabited key, I need insulin. I made a list of all the pharmacies and even endocrinologists who might have access to Insulin. I have a prescription on file at my local pharmacy, which can be transferred to whichever pharmacy I stumble upon.

The only problem is that the list I made is also at the bottom of the ocean. It is probably hospital time. Without phone or radio, the help of a stranger will be necessary.

I walk to the first beach house I find and knock. Or, really, I pound on that door with all the strength I have. I explain I am a type

1 diabetic who is without insulin and I am going to need a ride to the hospital to get some.

And all is good again. The next night I will probably run some other scenario in my head to put myself to sleep and continue to do the same thing every night until I leave, until I know I have thought about every possible scenario and, with a cool head, planned out what I would do.

WHY WE NEED TO FOCUS ON THE WHAT IF'S

Although we are quite capable of doing anything our hearts' desire, as adventurers with diabetes, we are at a higher risk if things go wrong. A normy, someone with a working pancreas, might be able to be stuck in the woods for ten days without food. But those same ten days for us, without food or insulin, would be devastating.

We need to make sure we are more prepared than the normies. We need to have a Plan B for when things go wrong. And then a Plan C for when Plan B fails. And a Plan D and Plan E...

Because the consequences are higher for us, we have to think about every possible thing that can go wrong when we put ourselves out in the elements. If we plan in the safety of our home, we can decide what the best course of action would be for each situation. We can with a cool, calm mind make decisions before the panic and fear sets in when things do go wrong.

We can also make preparations for any situation, like having two sources of insulin and keeping them in different locations, so if one location is compromised, we have a backup.

We should plan to have our paperwork in order to purchase more insulin from pharmacies if needed. We should know the locations of local hospitals and the procedures for calling 911 (or the equivalent) in foreign countries.

PLAN FOR THE WORST, BUT EXPECT THE BEST

Preparing like this makes it easier to have the confidence we need to bring diabetes into the wilderness. We may need to do more work ahead of time, but we can still do the same crazy things our adventure heroes do without ever letting diabetes become an excuse for not living out our dreams.

18

MANIPULATING FOR MAXIMUM MOTIVATION

Facebook, Instagram, and TikTok can be the ultimate time suck. You can scroll for hours through posts of food and cute kids from people you can barely remember.

But you can also make social media work for you. You can modify your timeline so that instead of sucking up your time with meaningless info, it will drip inspiration into your life.

It can become an environmental cue to change habits, just like we talked about in Chapter 12. Take the habit that you already may have, checking your Fsocial media page, and let it prompt you to refocus on adventure.

HOW TO MANIPULATE IT

First it might be a good idea to "Unfollow" anybody you don't actually know, like, and want to know more about. This doesn't mean you are "unfriending" them. You stay friends. They will never know you did this. It only means that their updates won't be cluttering your timeline.

When you find a post from them, simply click on the little arrow in the top, right corner, and click the Unfollow choice. Now you won't see any more posts from them in your timeline.

Next, find positive, inspirational pages to follow. This way, when you sit down to kill a few minutes, you find inspirational photos and great articles scrolling across your screen. Inspiration will now be seeking you out.

To start you out, I have listed ten terrific, inspirational pages to follow. Remember, if you want to continue seeing them in your timeline, click "like" or click on an article often to tell the Facebook wizards that you want to continue seeing these types of posts. You can also go on each page and after clicking like, click the following button and hit "See First" which will put it up higher and more frequently show in your feed and outsmart the algorithms.

You may want to start with the pages listed below, then go out and find your own inspirational pages.

You can do the same sort of thing with Instagram and TikTok, A link to all these pages can be found at SeaPeptide.com/aolinks.

COMPANIES

National Geographic Adventure- National Geographic ADVENTURE is for people who love outdoor activities and adventure travel. Its hallmarks are great writing from some of the best journalists working today, photography that stands firmly in the National Geographic tradition, and detailed guides that help readers plan and experience adventures of their own.

Adventure Journal- Adventure Journal is an online magazine—an independent voice for authentic outdoor adventure. World's #1 adventure blog, #2 cycling blog, #4 gear blog—according to Outside Magazine

Outside Magazine- A great magazine covering all types of adventures. Great gear reviews and ideas about places and sports I would never have thought of.

Matador Network- Matador is a global community of travel journalists, filmmakers, athletes, photographers, and writers producing original stories and videos on people, place, music, sports, and culture worldwide.

Intrepid Travel- We all travel for different reasons. People. Culture. Wildlife. Food. Landscapes. Cityscapes. Whatever motivates you, we're here to help you get stuck in.

GoPro- If you're looking for amazing pictures of people adventuring, this is the place to go. It both inspires me to adventure more and to learn to take better pictures.

Ocean Souls- Most of my adventures revolve around the ocean, so this one is a great source of inspiration. It consists mostly of beautiful photos of amazing places.

DIABETES PAGES

Beyond Type 1- Founded by some famous and truly talented people, Beyond Type 1 started as a very well designed Instagram campaign and eventually became a group that creates and funds a portfolio of programs, technologies and innovations that those living with Type 1 diabetes need to manage, live and thrive. Their goal is to highlight the brilliance of those fighting this disease every day while always working toward ensuring a cure is on its way.

Connected In Motion- Supports the active diabetes community through peer-led, outdoor adventure and sport programming. We are empowered by adventure.

Tandem Diabetes- Although technically a pump manufacturer, Tandem puts out a great Facebook page, highlighting interesting users and things going on in the diabetes world.

Dexcom- Dexcom CGM puts out interesting stories of people doing adventurous things while wearing a Dexcom.

PEOPLE

Dave Cornthwaite: Expedition 1000- Dave has traveled over

20,000 non-motorized miles in his adventures. He is in the midst of twenty-five different non-motorized travels of at least one thousand miles each. He's paddled theMississippi, skated across Australia, aquaskipped on the telly and taken one thousand photos in one thousand days, amongst other things.

Nomadic Matt's Travel Site- Learn how to make your dream trip a reality with daily tips, advice, and tricks on how to travel the world cheaper, smarter, and longer.

The Expeditioners- The Expeditioners comprises extreme photographers Roberto and Bella who traverse the world documenting their travels. From the most remote locations on the planet to the most luxurious hotels, come live a life that few ever do.

TripHackr- Specializing in Travel Hacking by providing the tools, reviews, and information you need to travel for less and maximize your trips around the world.

19

THE HAND YOU'VE BEEN DEALT

The first two days of my sailing adventure in Florida passed by without even a hint of a stiff breeze. They were sunny and warm, and I had hours and hours to enjoy the view and build my confidence with my new boat.

The third day could not have been any different. Overnight the winds had picked up so that, by 2 a.m., the sound of sailboat rigging banging against the mast woke me. I poked my head out of the cockpit of the boat to feel the still hot wind starting to blow with a vengeance.

By morning, it had solidified into a twenty-knot wind complete with a small craft advisory on the weather radio that I happened to miss that morning. I spent the day watching the storm clouds move in as I fought the wind and the waves it had whipped up overnight.

By noon, it was apparent that I had too much sail up, but I was too afraid to put a reef in the sail to decrease the size, since I had never done it before. The boat had become nearly impossible to manage in the storm that was brewing, which would have made that maneuver even harder.

After a gust of wind nearly knocked down my boat, I knew I was more afraid of capsizing than of reefing a sail and I got right to it.

Once I reduced the sail area, it became easier to sail my course to Hurricane Harbor at the close end of Key West. My plan was to stay there for the night and then, the next morning, sail around to Key West Harbor on the other side of the island to complete my 100-mile journey.

As I sat in port listening to the weather forecast for the next morning, the thought dawned on me I might not make my goal. The winds were expected to increase, as were the swells. After barely making it safely back to port that day, I wasn't about to go back out the next day to face even more weather.

I may have failed to make it 100-miles, but that wasn't truly my goal. My goal was to challenge myself, to see what I was made of. I wanted to test my fortitude to know how I would perform when things got scary. I wanted to have something to train for again.

And I did. I was proud of the decisions I made and how I held it together, much more than I would have completing the 100 miles under milder circumstances.

IT'S OK TO FAIL

Remember that the purpose of going out on these adventures is about finding the motivation to take our diabetes care to the next level. It is about broadening our worldview by going new places and experiencing new things. It is about choosing an athletic adventure that is big enough to inspire us.

And sometimes that means we will not finish what we set out to do. Especially when adventure depends on the weather or other things that are beyond your control, you cannot control your ability to succeed.

Maybe, if all the stars aligned and everything went according to plan, you could finish. But this world does not always go to plan. Things happen.

The weather turns nasty and you can't put in your last day of sailing. Or you have a series of horrible blood sugars that dehydrates you so much that you get serious calf cramps in the middle of your comeback triathlon. Or you get asthma so badly that you miss the last month of your training for a swim.

And sometimes, in adventuring, you will come home not finishing what was on your trail map. But that does not mean that you did not accomplish what you set out to accomplish.

Adventure is not about winning. It's about putting yourself out there and testing what you're made of. It's ok to fail on a course map as long as you don't fail in the real purpose of your adventure.

PLAY THE HAND YOU'VE BEEN DEALT

Everyone is given certain gifts and certain hurdles. Everyone has them. The best you can do in this world is to play the hand you've been dealt. You have diabetes and that means it may jump out at you at the totally wrong moment.

A really bad low five minutes before the start of a game. A flu that turns into a never ending high that turns into a hospital stay the week before you leave.

The more time and emotion you waste on getting pissed off, the less you will have to persevere. Those are just the cards you've been dealt. Play them. And play them well. Don't judge yourself by anyone else's standards. Make the most of every opportunity and every ability you have.

And then celebrate the hell out of the fact that you are out doing much more than 99% of this world that is too focused on what they can't do instead of what they can do.

20

COMMIT AND GO PUBLIC

When I started planning my first adventure, the 100-mile sail, I spent months detailing my course, deciding what to bring, and dreaming about how great it would feel to be alone on a boat for four days. But at some point, the trip had to go from planning to doing. I needed to commit.

That moment came when I pushed "buy" on my non-refundable airplane ticket. It took every bit of birthday money and Christmas money that I had to purchase that ticket, and, once I did, there was no going back.

COMMIT

There comes a time in every journey when it changes from dreaming and planning to executing. At some point in the near future, you are going to have to commit to this project.

For some people that has to do with laying out non-refundable monies to book the trip. For others, it is finally telling the one person who will be affected most by the trip, whether that is a spouse, kids, parents, or boss. But, in order to make this dream a reality, you have to commit.

AND GO PUBLIC

Another major turning point in my trip was when I told friends, family, and strangers through my blog that I was going. That kind of public announcement gave me a sense of accountability. I certainly didn't want to flake on myself, but having to tell everyone else I knew, that I couldn't hack it, just wasn't an option.

There's another reason that at some point in this process you should go public. When you share your adventure with other people, it inspires them. Watching a person who is just like them, stepping out of their comfort zone and into the wild challenges them. Your excitement will wear off on them. They will see how this adventure has given you the motivation to take better care of your health, and they might want that for themselves.

There is no need to keep all of this to yourself if, by sharing, you can help so many other people with very little extra work.

HOW TO SHARE

Some of you may be experts at sharing every little detail of your lives with other people. You may even be one of those who tends to overshare. Or you might be a person who takes a lot of cajoling to share about your adventure. Whatever type of person you naturally are, it is time to stretch yourself to share the benefits of adventure with those in your circle of influence.

So, how do you do this most effectively? It starts with the small things. Share your intentions to adventure on your social networks like Twitter, Facebook, Instagram, or whatever other platform you use. And don't just share that you are going on a trip. Share the benefits of how it is helping to motivate you to take better care of your health.

You may even want to start a blog, a place where you can share your stories of planning and training for your adventure. It may even help to keep you accountable to the process, sharing details of your ups and downs of adventuring.

And when you are finally on your adventure, take us with you. Post tons of photos and videos. Let us know about every beautiful and strange and amazing part of your journey.

By sharing your story, your adventure will not only serve to benefit you, but, also, the hundreds, or maybe even thousands, of people within your sphere of influence.

SO...

WHAT NOW?

Congratulations!!! You have officially finished Adventure On. I hope your enthusiasm is even stronger now than it was then. I'm sure you have made some pretty big changes to your life and how you take care of your health.

So, now what?

Well, first off, don't let this just be another program you read through and do nothing about. If you don't already have a firm adventure on the books you are currently training for, go back over each of the Chapters. Study them and take the time to put into practice each step we went over.

Now is the time to pat yourself on the back! Throw yourself a little party with a big group of friends or reward yourself with a little something like a new pair of running socks or a nice dinner out. Find some way to congratulate yourself. You have taken the first critical steps to changing the way you view diabetes and who you are as an adventurer.

Now, is also the time to reevaluate your progress towards your adventure and to remind yourself of all the wonderful things you learned over the course of the book

How are your plans going? Do you have a firm adventure in mind? Do you have a training plan in place? Have you been trying to implement the "Just 1% Better" mentality?

Have you been changing the stories you tell yourself about who you are and what you are capable of? Have you been freaking out? I know I have.

Have you been reading and watching inspirational books, movies, and Facebook posts? Have you been taking real, actual steps towards making your dream adventure a reality?

If your plans aren't solid just yet, why don't you go back through some of the old chapters and refresh your memory a bit. Maybe something will jump out at you this time that you didn't see the first time around.

Take some time this week to build on your adventure plans, to make them a little more solid. Actually, decide on a block of time to spend planning your adventure and write it in your schedule.

Don't let anything get in your way. Remember, the time you spend on yourself will pay off for everyone around you when you have more energy and you are healthier.

If you need answers or encouragement, remember that you have full access to the Adventure On Community for as long as you would like. Use it. Post your questions. Ask for encouragement. And take the time to answer a few questions from your fellow adventurers. Maybe the only encouragement you need is to be reminded that you hold a vast amount of knowledge that could be helpful to another person just starting out on this journey.

I would love to hear about your plans, too. Feel free to email me at erin@seapeptide.com with your plans or any comments or questions you have.

Now get ready to see, firsthand, what adventure will do to your life. I can't wait to see all the pictures and videos of your next adventure!!!

Read on for a sneak peek of
CALIFORNIA PROMISES!!!

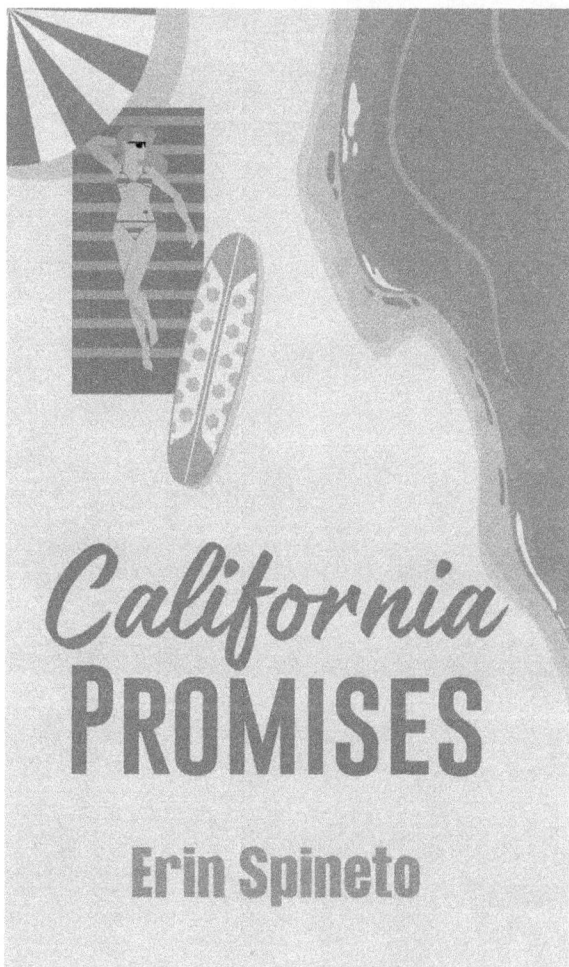

California
PROMISES

Erin Spineto

If you're looking for fiction with a strong female
character with diabetes, read on for an excerpt from
California Promises, a friends-to-lovers RomCom.

1

CHARLIE

Tomboy. The expression is a cheap shot, a jab at a girl's ability to play the Feminine Game. But, in that word, I've found my hidden superpower. The freedom to peek behind the fortifications of Guyland, to discover the side they'd never show a "real" girl.

Of course, that label also means that I can't use any of that insight to find a man of my own since no worthwhile guy in his right mind would date a tomboy.

A text flashes on my phone next to a picture of Principal Dick Vernon from The Breakfast Club.

Glenn: Need Confirmation by Tomorrow!

I don't know why I ever surrendered this number to Glenn Kratzcy, the man in charge at Big&Lime, the tech startup I slave for. Though, at a super-juvenile twenty-nine, I'm not sure he can be called a man. Maybe the under-ripe chief of a band of milk-fed imbeciles?

Another message lights up my screen.

Glenn: Dirk is going to take the lead on pushing ahead with the reminder app that he proposed at our last meeting.

That he proposed? Glenn actually thinks Dirk's mansplaining my proposal in our last meeting was him coming up with it.

Beyond the computer on my bedroom desk, out the row of wood-framed windows, is a sky painted with giant swaths of neon pink and purple, fading into a darkening navy opposite the sun as she waves goodbye before slipping beneath the saltwater.

The hot cyan skies that bled into my upstairs bedroom when I sat down at my computer this afternoon have drifted off without my notice. I've been entrenched in trying to "work the problem." Though I only proposed Nudge to Big&Lime this week, I've been developing the project for years.

My phone buzzes again. God, I hate every-sentence-texters.

Glenn: We think Dirk has the best perspective and familiarity with the subject to guide the project in the right direction. I want you to work with him on it.

I pound out my reply.

Charlie: Perspective and familiarity? You mean he has a cock. Because that's the obvious prerequisite for knowing anything about sports or fitness. Forget the fact that the app was my creation or the fact that I have played more ball than he ever has, unless, of course, you count playing with his own marble sack. He is male, so, obviously, he's the one you put in charge.

Rereading what would be my resignation, I slam it down on my charcoal-stained desk. I need this job, no matter what kind of misogynistic quips I have to put up with.

"I, I love the colorful clothes she wears, And the way the sunlight plays upon her hair," the Beach Boys tune wafting in through my open window entices me from this funk and towards a party mood, but I have to stop this Kamikaze flight before it tanks my future at Bad&Lime.

My phone blares again.

Seriously, Glenn? For a tech genius, you sure don't grasp texting.

Glenn: Let me know ASAP. Dirk is going to start work tomorrow at first light.

Of course, that asshat would go in early Saturday to hijack my baby.

Working with Dirk is a total shitfest, but enduring it means Nudge would exist in the real world. How cool would that be? Something I've been working on for years, helping people.

To bring it there, though, I would have to work with that troglodyte every day for months. I'm not sure I could take the constant stream of douchey humor without going all "bitch mode" as they call it.

"*I'm picking up good vibrations, She's giving me excitations,*" the song continues.

"Charlie! Get down here. And put on your dancing shoes, pronto."

I lay my hands on dingy white paint covering the window sill and peer over them. On the weathered deck below, my roommate, Indigo dances wildly to the music that's been breezing in my window.

Erasing my last text, I slip the phone into my pocket. I wonder if Greyson has shown up, yet. He always gets my head spinning in the right direction.

I drift over to the walk-in closet I share with my roommate, Bex, though share is an overstatement. Bex has allocated a quarter of the space for storage of my limited wardrobe and paltry shoe selection. The other three-quarters houses her extensive clothing collection.

My dirty blue and white checkerboard Vans in front of the closet stare at me. These are not dancing shoes. Tonight's a Fancy Vans kind of night.

My Fancy Vans aren't your normal everyday shoes. They are the color of Napili Bay at the west end of Maui and made from the softest canvas I have ever touched. When I slip them on, they lend me a twinge of confidence and a snippet of joy.

Toiling non-stop in the cramped bedroom all afternoon, I've shed most my clothes. Since no one would appreciate me coming downstairs in my cutoffs and an old sports bra, I slip on a white tank-top with random flecks of aqua to match my dancin' shoes and toss a blue and black checked flannel over it. I take out my ponytail, bleached the lightest shade of blond from too many hours in the salt water, and run my fingers through my hair. Good enough.

Pausing for just a moment at the top of the stairs, I rehearse my opening lines. Smile. "Hi. How are you involved with the film? How do you know Indigo?"

Small talk with large groups of new people has always been difficult. I am way more at home in small groups, but I work hard not to show it. I've found that a couple of opening lines are all I need. Once I get people talking about themselves, I don't have to do much more than listen.

Downstairs, I search for Greyson in the throng of people filling the dated kitchen of our beach shack. Unrecognizable bodies fill the seats at the handmade table in the adjoining dining room and pour out onto the deck and further onto the sand.

Our shack was built in the 1930s in the side yard of a beach-front mansion in Del Mar, California, the same strip of land that hosts the multi-million-dollar homes of Bill Gates, Theodor Geisel, and half of the current NFL and MLB stars when they're not killing it on the field. It was designed for the original owner as a workshop to shape surfboards.

In the '60s, the new owner converted it into a guest house with a kitchen, dining room, and small living room downstairs, two tiny bedrooms upstairs, and the most glorious back deck I have ever seen. It hangs over the sand with the surf only sixty yards from its back railing.

It hasn't been updated since the '60s and it shows in the chipped exterior, faulty plumbing, and noises it makes with every step, but moving into the dilapidated bungalow with Indigo and Bex means I can write 2830 Ocean Front as my address.

Ocean. Front.

Every morning I eat breakfast and drink my first Diet Dr Pepper of the day with my feet buried in the dew-drenched sand. Each night, while I drift off to sleep, I listen to the sound of waves dancing on the shore. And at night, as I slumber, the salt air invades my dreams and draws me away to islands filled with warm uncrowded surf, boundless tropical fruit, and dazzling golden sunshine.

Tonight Indigo is hosting a party for the cast and crew of the third indie film she wrote, produced, and directed solo. Later on, she'll show the movie on the giant screen anchored at the edge of the deck.

I make my way through the crowd of Victoria's Secret model

wannabes to the cooler and pop out the Diet Dr Pepper Indigo hid for me under the bottles of Stone and Lagunitas beer. I hadn't known Indigo when I moved in a few months ago, but she has tuned in to my habits faster than most people I've met.

I quickly pour the soda into a pint glass so some cheesy dude doesn't come up with the bright idea to ask me the oh-so-clever and super-insulting, "So why aren't you drinking tonight? You get too wild when you do?" Nothing makes me want to jump in bed faster than a sleazy pickup line.

Trying to shift mental gears, I meander to the splintered railing. Indigo has strung what must be hundreds of tiny white lights in the Banyan tree, their light pouring over the railing and out onto the sand. She is always telling me how superb lighting can change a scene, and tonight she has set the stage for a celebration worthy of her accomplishment.

"How are you ever going to entice a man in those sorry excuses for shoes?" Bex yelps so the guy she's been eye-banging won't hold my appearance against her.

Bexley Liddell isn't naturally pretty, with legs too short to be considered sexy and a face too forgettable to make up for it. But she does know how to maximize what little she has. She's a whiz with makeup and only wears what will show off her well-earned bum. After ninety minutes of preening and painting, she'll turn every guy's head with the sheer volume of hotness she's able to amass.

"Because that is my goal in life, Bex," sarcasm dripping from my lips.

I appraise her victim for the night. He's not a bad choice, wavy blond hair probably styled with the salt from a surf earlier, shoulders hardened by years of paddling. Maybe I should give Bex's shoe theory a try if it could win me a guy like that.

"So I have decided on our Summer Goal," she exclaims gleefully without taking her eyes off Surfer Boy.

Bex and I have been friends since we were seven, and every year since we had a Summer Goal. Bex would come up with a goal by the last day of school and we would devise our battle plan at my house on the first night of summer. I think it was a way to distract herself from the dark void her father left when he bailed on seven-year-old Bexley, and the overbearing shadow her mom radiated when demanding Bex behave the way a proper lady should, withdrawing her love when she didn't comply.

When we were eight, our objective was to ride our bikes to the store every single day for a triple-decker scoop of ice cream at Thrifty's. At ten, we reached for the heavens and attempted to dip our feet in the ocean each and every day.

By the time we were twelve, our focus shifted. That summer our target was Timothy and Michael Holmes, the cutest twins in our grade. It didn't matter to Bex that I was more interested in Bryce Taylor; the only acceptable goal that summer was to date twins.

She developed a three-pronged plan. First, we had to become as thin and tan as possible. For Bex, that meant counting every calorie that passed her lips and loafing in the sun for hours on end. For me, that meant surfing every morning while she was still snoozing.

The second part was to ride our matching, yellow cruisers past their spectacular, two-story home every day in our cutest cutoffs and bikini tops, hoping they would invite us in. For the last step, Bex would orchestrate a game of Spin-The-Bottle, decrying, "All boys can be swayed with a steamy kiss."

A spark of hope at what this summer could bring lights my chest. "Summer Goal Number Nineteen. It better be a good one."

Bex tears her eyes off her man, grabs my hands, and bounces with anticipation. "I am so super excited about this one, Charlie."

I try to match her elation, but that level of girliness is hard to mimic. "Okay, Bex. Hit me."

"So, this summer, I am going to find us boyfriends so we can both be married by spring and then start having matching babies that can totally grow up together."

Her hands flit all over the place, emphasizing each and every point. "And we have to make sure our men like each other so we can take family vacations and barbecue in our backyard."

"Our Backyard? We're gonna share a house with our broods?" I laugh.

Logic is not Bex's strong suit. That was always my part--

to figure out the details--taking her crazy ideas and developing rational plans to bring them to fruition.

"No, dummy. You'll live in the house directly in back of us and we can rip down the fence in between so we can share a yard and your kids can swim in the pool that my independently wealthy husband will have custom-designed for me."

Bex may be my polar opposite, but she's great at noticing my weaknesses and pushing me to work on them, like my lack of drive to find a husband. Over the years, I've become a better version of myself because of it.

"And all this is going to happen this summer?" I take a sip of my soda. "You can just will it to happen?"

"Looks like I already did." She nods towards her Surfer Boy, now talking to an equally hot friend. "Remember not to settle on either one too soon, just in case the one with the long hair is into me. You know how I love long hair. And best friends never take each other's sloppy seconds."

With that, she drags me towards Step One of the plan.

"So what's your deal?" the brunette one says to me, his efforts focused on his consolation prize now that he lost his battle for Bex's attention to his long-haired friend.

"My deal?" I shoot back hoping for a better question. Of course, I'm stuck with the champion conversationalist.

"Yeah. Like, what do you do? What're you looking for? What turns you on?"

I put on my best ditsy accent. "Well, like, for fun I drink. And I totally love to conversate. And boys turn me on. What about you?"

Waiting for him to catch on is an exercise in futility. Dopey perks up and hums, "You turn me on."

I glance over my shoulder hoping Greyson will come save me from this disaster.

Bex considers the gaping smile on Predictable Boy's face and gives my arm a squeeze of approval. If only she knew.

After a lifetime of vapid questions from the boys, stellar flirting from Bex, and what can hardly be called proficient flirting from me, I've had enough. I excuse myself to grab another drink, but with Bex hanging on both boys now, they don't miss me.

Leaning on the wobbly railing, the salt air from the water playing in the darkness beyond the reach of our deck comforts me. What I wouldn't give to pick up a board and be out there now instead of trying to play nice with a bunch of strangers. And making my current social stress worse, deciphering the predicament at work is diverting my mental energy from pretending to enjoy small talk.

"I just met the man I'm going to marry," squeals the leader of the throng of girls behind me. "He has the most beautiful blue eyes that just sing out that you are the only woman for him. He has super thick brown hair and the perfect stubble," she says motioning to each body part like her friends have no clue where his hair or eyes or stubble go.

"And he is totally ripped, biceps as big as my head, and a shoulder tattoo, which is, like, totally my favorite."

A grip of nooowaaay's and ohmygaaaawd's ring out like the squawking of seagulls.

"He bumped into me inside, and he looks deep into my eyes, so my heart, like, almost stops, and then, after he touches my arm, he says, 'Sorry about that babe. I didn't see you there, but I do now.' But. He. Does. Now," she proclaims punctuating each word with a bob of her head.

I scan the crowd for the man they've all been oohing and ahhing over; that 'But I do now' line sounds familiar.

"Briiiiiii. You are so lucky!!!" I swear they all cry in unison.

"And get this, he's a fireman. A real-life freakin' hero fireman."

And, at that, I know Greyson's here.

Greyson Steele and I have been friends since I was fifteen when his cousin invited him to hang with our group of friends during our regular Friday Night Pizza and Bowling.

He had the same effect on the girls back then, too. I hate to admit it, but even I was drawn in for a hot minute. I'm not usually a masochist; I don't enter fights I can't win, and I cannot win any girly competition.

I watched from a distance as he navigated the crush of girls fawning all over him while we ordered. I grabbed my cup and filled it up with Dr Pepper and slid into the large round booth at the far end of the restaurant like we did every Friday night. The girls were buzzing around, waiting until Greyson chose a seat so they could dive into the booth after him to monopolize his attention, until the strangest thing happened.

He walked over to where I was sitting at the edge of the booth and said, "Wanna slide over?"

Dirty looks exploded from the girls signifying their plans to get a leg up in this game had just been thwarted by the girl they didn't even consider competition. For a brief moment, I thought a guy actually chose me over a mob of girls way prettier and certainly more well-versed in the art of flirting. Don't worry, though, it didn't last long.

A few minutes later he leaned over, motioning like he wanted to tell me something. Only me. I leaned in, awaiting the sweet secret, and he whispers, "You remind me of my sister."

Gravity concentrated beneath me drawing me back into my seat. It only took him ten minutes to figure me out.

I was defeated, but at least he saved me the embarrassment of flinging myself at him before he realized he would never want a girl who can out-surf him, out-think him, and who probably spent way less time getting ready than he did.

Although I didn't win the girly showdown that night, I walked away with a much better prize--Greyson Steele as my best friend.

Finish reading CALIFORNIA PROMISES now! Get your copy at bit.ly/CaProm2

SNEEK PEEK OF ISLANDS AND INSULIN!!

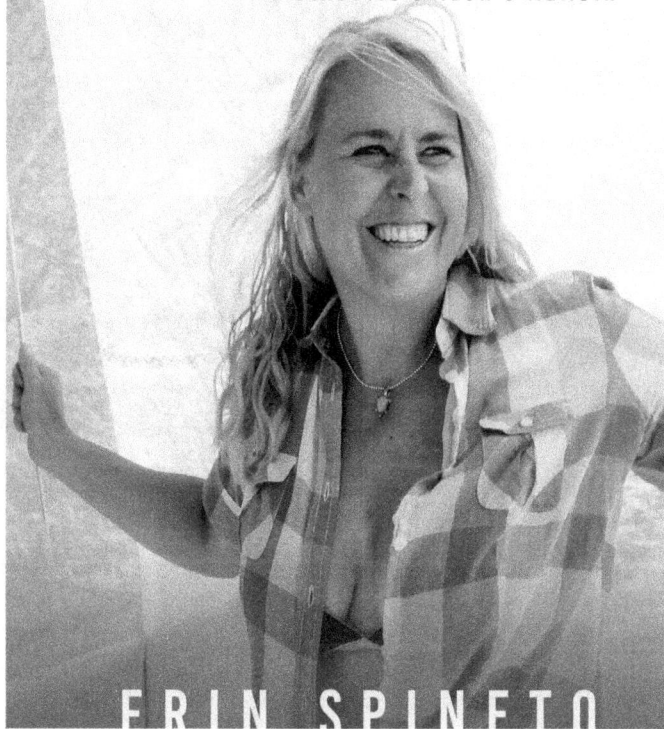

""Erin Spineto should be proud as hell for being it, living it, and writing it."
--Kerri Sparling, creator and author of Six Until Me

ISLANDS
AND
INSULIN
A DIABETIC SAILOR'S MEMOIR

ERIN SPINETO

Love stories of adventure? Want to read about Erin's maiden voyage? Read on for a sample of Islands and Insulin: A Diabetic Sailor's Memoir!

1

It's past seven on a Friday night and the streets of Balboa Island, once jammed with people enjoying the summer beach scene, are now shimmering from a recent downpour and devoid of any signs of life.

Tony and I just drove down Pacific Coast Highway from my parents' home in Seal Beach where Shea and Eli are safely tucked into bed under the watchful eye of their Nana and Moe.

We are meeting another couple for dinner and we all arrive at exactly the same moment, a good five minutes before we agreed to meet. We meet up in the crosswalk of the empty, rain-soaked street and exchange hugs, handshakes, and a few "good to see you agains" before realizing that maybe we shouldn't be standing in the middle of the street.

As we make our way to the restaurant, Hank reaches down for the hand of the girl that is usually there, without realizing that the person beside him now is Tony. A little awkward for two guys who are only in the same place because I invited them both to come.

The last time those boys were in the same room was at Tony's and my wedding over a decade ago. Hank didn't know Pam back then. She had come on the scene recently, and tonight was the first time I would get to meet her.

I had read plenty about her in the emails I received from Hank over the years and knew she had to be a great gal to put up with him, but I am a little nervous about all of us being able to have a good time tonight.

The empty streets make for an empty restaurant and, except for a large group over in the corner, we have the place to ourselves. We dive into some small talk, catching up mostly, the sort of light conversation you can get through while you're really focusing on how different everyone looks.

Older, maybe.

Like the people I used to watch on TV sitcoms as a kid, the ones who played the adults. Hank and Tony and Pam all look like those adults to me. I don't know why it surprises me. We are all in our mid-thirties.

But it does surprise me; it must mean I look like an adult to them too, even though I feel nothing like it. Hank runs his hand over his neatly shorn hair and reassures me that I haven't aged a day since high school. "Except your hands," he adds. "They look old."

"Gee, thanks," I say giving them a good once-over.

It was just last week that I realized my hands started to look like my mother's. I remember how they looked when she would read to me before my nap and I would watch her hands as she turned the pages. Many years at the beach wrinkled them beyond her age.

Thirty-four years in the sun has aged my hands, too, and I wonder if my kids think the same thing as I read to them each night before bed.

The waitress interrupts our pleasantries to take our drink order. The boys' banter about the beers and Pam decides on some wine. I go with the old reliable diet soda.

Hank makes sure to get the waitress' name and flirt a bit, a classic Hank move, but tonight it is performed with more subtlety than when he was younger. A bit more charm and a little less player. The years have tempered his wily ways.

I look over to see how Pam reacts; many a girl has been greatly offended by Hank's gregarious ways. She tucks her short blond hair behind her ear and just rolls her eyes, slightly amused. I like this girl already.

When we were younger, Hank acted as a filter for new people we would meet. If they could put up with his antics and even enjoy them a bit, I knew I would get along with them. Those who were offended or irritated usually didn't end up making the shortlist of great people IN my life. It was an easy litmus test for new acquaintances.

Pam just might make that shor list if she continues being so laid back.

"I'm glad I rode this morning," Tony says looking over the outrageous calorie count on the menu. Tony is twelve weeks into a sixteen-week training program for the Oceanside Half Ironman Triathlon, scheduled just one month from tonight. "Biking sixty miles makes it really easy to justify food like this."

"So what kind of bike do you ride?" Hank asks.

I am relieved they found something to talk about. Having to carry the conversation scared me and seeing that I'm quiet by nature, it would have made for a dull evening.

The boys drift off into talk of Sram this and Zipp that. Pam appears to be as bored by cycling conversation as I am. We get into the usual stuff girls talk about when they are starting to get to know each other. She complains of her house being too small, of her and Hank deciding if they should renovate their duplex into one big house for the both of them. Hank has enough clothes to fill a bedroom.

"I don't even have a real closet. All of my stuff is in one of those freestanding wardrobes." Hank chimes in.

"Just don't go too big," I say. "We just moved into a bigger place and it takes two hours to clean. It's way too big. I would so much rather clean the seven hundred square feet we used to live in, not that I really do much of the cleaning anyways."

"You must do the cooking, then?" Pam asks.

"No. Tony does most of the cooking. He's a trained chef so he thinks my cooking sucks."

"Well, then, what do you have to offer?" she asks.

"Pam," Hank chides her.

It's weird to see him with Pam in that way, taking care of her and feeling responsible for who she is. It's that sort of relationship when you're with someone for such a long time and you see their behavior as a reflection of yourself.

He is worried that she might offend me, which is odd because he has never worried about offending me himself. I suppose he just wants me to like her as much as I want him to like Tony.

I don't mind her question, though. Her frankness is refreshing. I prefer transparent people who will be rude if it's what they're thinking, much more than people who only tell you what they think you want to hear. I could go the rest of my life and die happy without being told one more time what someone thinks I want to hear.

"I don't know what I have to offer," I say laughing.

"So, how was that sailing trip of yours?" Hank asks, trying to change the topic.

I try to think of a way to take five days of adventure and put it simply into one sentence. Luckily, the waitress walks up with our pizza in a heavy cast iron pan and sets it on the table giving me a few moments to think. She takes the spatula and serves us each a piece before walking away to grab another round of drinks.

"I've never been more scared in my life," I say.

The beeping coming from my back pocket pulls me away for a moment. I check my phone which is silent and then reach for the continuous glucose monitor in my other pocket. It reads out my blood sugar at the moment, 385.

"Shit," I mutter to myself.

I retrieve the insulin pump hooked to my belt to give myself a big dose of insulin to fix the problem. At least, it wasn't the nerves that killed my appetite.

I look up and notice everyone at the table is still waiting for me to finish my answer. From the look on Pam's face, I realize I have totally freaked her out. No one has told her yet that I am a diabetic.

"All I know is there's no way in Hell I should have been out there like that."

6 APRIL 1996
LA JOLLA, CA

I close my eyes and I can still see that moment years before when it all changed. It's as clear as yesterday, and yet it seems a lifetime away. The symptoms were there, but they weren't anything I really paid any attention to.

Being only nineteen, I was not tuned in to what my body was trying to tell me. My time was spent ditching college classes and surfing and hanging out with friends.

I was never one to drink water, never really liked the taste. Apple juice, chocolate milk, Dr Pepper, now those were worthy of drinking. Water just seemed like a waste of time.

But I started drinking it by the boatload, craving it really. I couldn't sit through a Physics lecture without getting up at least three times to drink from the fountain (this was in the days before carrying a PBA-free water bottle everywhere was in fashion).

With all the extra water came all the extra bathroom trips. At least, that's what I thought was causing my nocturnal wanderings towards the toilet. I tried to explain it away. It's just the heat. It was spring and the weather was heating up.

As I got up for the third time to miss yet another section of the lecture, and was forced to drink out of that overused, under-cleaned shiny metal box of cooled tap water, I told myself the lecture was just really boring and I was looking for a way to stay awake.

Physics was my favorite subject though, so I don't know how I convinced myself of that one. Maybe it was just the best explanation I could come up with at the time.

To make matters worse, I was studying for finals in the thick of it all. I spent one evening with my roommate, Martha, at the food court on campus so that we would have easy access to the soda machine while we studied. I never developed a taste for coffee, so my study drink of choice was Dr Pepper. I must have had about eight, twenty-ounce drinks that night.

And that wasn't Diet. Diet was for fools.

It was all real for me.

After studying that night, I couldn't find a way to slow down to get some rest. I lay in that state between awake and asleep when thoughts run amok and you can't control them and you can only sit and watch them run all over the place and make no sense at all.

My dreams that night were filled with Organic Chemistry equations. The kind where two types of molecules in their 3-D structure are blended into an entirely new molecule. They were converting over and over again in front of me, taunting me with every conversion.

I assumed the insomnia was due to stress and finals. The minor symptoms I was feeling didn't register as the beginnings of anything serious until I was riding my bike home from school the next week and came to Hell Hill.

Most of my runs and bike rides ended on this shady, tree-lined hill. It was only about a quarter-mile long, but the incline made it a challenge. My goal each day was to ride to the top without being forced to stand up on the pedals. At the time I was in good shape and was making it to the top fairly consistently.

But not that day.

Halfway up the hill, I was so weak and light-headed that I was forced to get off my bike and sit down for a few minutes. Normally it would have taken me less than two minutes to get home from that point. Thirty-five minutes later I was still trying to get there.

I had to lean all of my weight on the bike to wheel my failing body home, stopping every few hundred feet to gather more strength. When I got home I sat on the couch dazed while my roommates tried to help. Martha came in first.

"Erin, you feeling alright?"

In the spring of 1996, La Jolla was the perfect backdrop for a wonderfully easy life. My parents were still footing the bill while I made my way through school. Classes were easy and the beach was close by.

In my last three years at the University of California, San Diego, I shared a three-story condo with six girls. Each year we had a different group of girls paying the rent. Every summer some of the girls would move out and new ones would move in, which made it the perfect place for me.

With that many people coming and going I could stay unnoticed, well-hidden. Martha was the only girl to live with me for all three years and one of the only ones who didn't let me fade entirely into the background. She was consistent and reliable, not one to add drama to any situation.

"I don't know," I tried to answer. She sat down beside me trying to assess the situation.

"What happened?"

I did my best to relay the story in my confused state.

"Maybe you were just working out too hard. Here have some licorice; maybe you just need some sugar."

If she only knew that sugar was exactly what was killing me. I recovered after about an hour and moved on. I spent the next few days trying to explain away what happened. I was sick a week before. I wasn't a hundred percent yet. I went too hard too soon.

I had no idea it was really the diabetes starting to show itself.

Finish reading Islands and Insulin today at bit.ly/IslandInsulin

Sign up now for the Salties Scoop at bit.ly/SPSscoop
to get exclusive release info, bonus scenes and epilogues,
a secret look into Erin's life, and so much more!

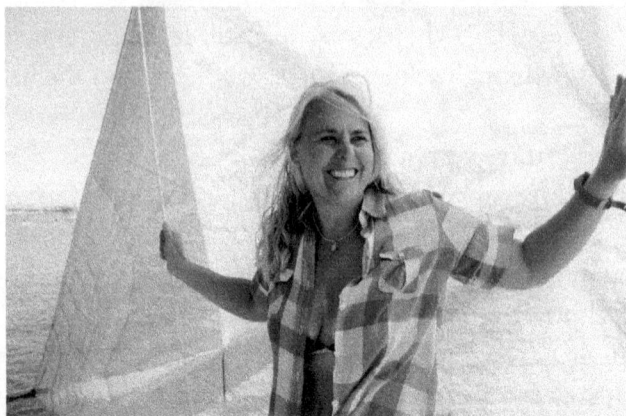

ABOUT THE AUTHOR

Erin Spineto started her writing journey in 2011 with Islands and Insulin, her memoir of sailing solo 100 miles down the Florida Keys with type 1 diabetes back in a time when doctors were foolish enough to recommend against this kind of wild adventure with diabetes.

Since then she has moved on to fiction and is currently working on Warrior Women, a three-book angsty RomCom series full of female surfers who happen to have diabetes and other autoimmune issues.

Erin's journey with autoimmune conditions started in 1996 with type 1 diabetes. She added hyperthyroidism to the mix in 2007, and has rounded out her collection with a little Anti-Synthetase Syndrome.

Not letting anything slow her down, Erin is also a long-distance endurance adventurer and autoimmune advocate who uses stories to encourage others with chronic illness to go big.

Erin started surfing at age five when she stood up on her boogie board and realized waves were so much more fun to ride standing up. Since then she has had a love affair with empty beaches, warm water, and a post-surf lunch of fish tacos and Diet Dr Pepper (though she's had to give that up to fight the ASS) eaten on a patio in the sun with her own real life hero, Tony, and their two surfing teenagers.

CONNECT WITH ME

I would love to continue this conversation. You can read all about all of my adventures past and present, as well as read about my thoughts on diabetes and adventure on my website, SeaPeptide.com.

You can connect with me:
On Instagram: Instagram.com/erinspineto
On Facebook: Facebook.com/erinspinetoauthor
On Twitter: Twitter.com/erinspineto

I would love to hear about your adventures. you can email me at erin@seapeptide.com or tag some of your own adventure photos with #seapeptideadventures. I look for these often.

www.ingramcontent.com/pod-product-compliance
Lightning Source LLC
Chambersburg PA
CBHW030253030426
42336CB00009B/369